*f*P

Between Expectations

Lessons from a Pediatric Residency

MEGHAN MACLEAN WEIR, MD

Free Press
New York London Toronto Sydney

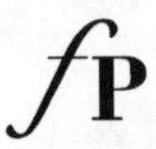

Free Press
A Division of Simon & Schuster, Inc.
1230 Avenue of the Americas
New York, NY 10020

First Free Press hardcover edition March 2011

Jill Putorti

Manufactured in the United States of America

10 9 8 7 6 5 4 3 2 1

Library of Congress Cataloging-in-Publication Data

Weir, Meghan MacLean.
Between expectations: lessons from a pediatric residency / Meghan MacLean Weir.
p.; cm.
Includes bibliographical references.
1. Weir, Meghan MacLean. 2. Children's Hospital (Boston, Mass.). 3. Pediatricians—Massachusetts—Boston—Biography. 4. Residents (Medicine)—Massachusetts—Boston—Biography. I. Title.
[DNLM: 1. Weir, Meghan MacLean. 2. Children's Hospital (Boston, Mass.). 3. Pediatrics—Personal Narratives. WZ 100 W425 2011]
RJ43.W45A3 2011
618.9200092—dc22
[B] 2010024628

ISBN 978-1-4391-8908-5
ISBN 978-1-4391-8909-2 (ebook)

For Gus

To be allowed to witness is a holy and incredible gift.

Randolph L. Markey

Contents

Between Expectations

Prologue

On the last day before our residency officially starts, when we are still playing at being doctors, before the decisions are actually placed in our hands, four of us from our intern class of more than forty stand close together during rounds in the neonatal intensive care unit (NICU). We watch as newborns are discussed in a jumble of numbers and words that are at times indecipherable. We cringe while last year's interns, just one day short of becoming juniors, are grilled without reprieve by the attending physician, being made to defend each of the myriad of decisions that had been made overnight. I listen, not with the growing sense of terror I had anticipated, but with a dullness that tamps down all possibility of visceral response. I am quiet, within and without, and inconspicuous in a way I have never before wanted to be.

It is only because I have become a shadow that I continue to breathe evenly when the alarm bells go off. I do not perspire; my heart does not race. I listen calmly as voices are raised and the orderly collection of doctors and nurses begins to buzz with activity. They say things that I don't understand, but there are also phrases that manage to penetrate: "twenty-five-week triplets" and "as many hands as we can get" and "come with me." Only after we have been thrown into motion do I realize they intend for us to assist at this delivery of squirming infants who are about to be born more than three months too soon.

We had all been trained for this scenario, in theory, with textbooks boasting glossy colored photos, in classrooms without air conditioning, each of us in turn taking hold of the various instruments—bag and mask, laryngoscope, and finally endotracheal tubes—that would be provided at the deliveries where resuscitation was called for. We were drilled and we were timed. Still, what was so markedly absent from all these demonstrations was the mother and her child.

Only Laura knew what such a birth would smell of: the blood and sweat and desperation filling a room that had housed so many similar scenes before, at once detracting from and amplifying the singularity of how a family can materialize as if from nothing, of how small miracles occur. Maybe this was why she ran with such determination and authority, or maybe it was simply because—as I was to learn later on in the year—she was so brave.

Then we are in a stairwell, just us four, trailing behind Alli, an arresting almost junior resident with the sort of dimples that should make her incapable of intimidation, but of whom I am (in that moment) completely terrified. We run full tilt behind her, not knowing where these stairs lead but understanding that somewhere there will be a door that will open onto surgeons and a woman who has three babies on the way.

Of our group of four interns, only Laura had rotated through the neonatal intensive care unit during medical school. Perhaps that is why she so easily keeps pace with Alli, having at least some vague idea of what awaits and what becomes expected when an infant comes into the world far too soon. Perhaps she had even, in another hospital and in a vastly different role, been handed such a child, its small, slick body finding the curve of her arms beneath the sterile pink and blue hospital towels, its lips parting to shriek heartily in protest or else whimper softly in a cry so weak that a mask was quickly placed over its mouth to help it breathe.

I am behind Neil and Kate. For some reason that I cannot explain, my hand has found the center of Kate's back, is resting just beneath her shoulder blades as we clump together, slowing down to take a turn on a landing, and I move it from side to side, stroking her in a gesture of reassurance. Later she tells me, "You were so sweet, rubbing my back."

I am embarrassed because we are still new to this hospital and to each other, so I dismiss the moment, laughing: "I wasn't rubbing your back. I was pushing you in front of me."

We are able to laugh like this now, because Alli had turned to Neil, stopping us on the final landing of the stairwell, and held out a laryngoscope, the blade closed and flat against the handle but still gleaming and somehow sinister in the yellow lights. She had stopped suddenly, causing Kate and me to bump up against each other while perched several stairs above them. Laura had kept going and overshot the scene that we looked down on.

"Have you ever used one of these before?" Alli asks Neil then, offering the blade again, thrusting it forward into the space between them.

Neil shrugs, at a loss as to how to find the right balance of reassuring competence and honesty. I had always imagined that there should be a single moment, a crossing over of boundaries, a definition of self. On the one side of this line there is childhood, a red tricycle with yellow handlebar streamers and your mother's hands on a long white kitchen countertop covered with flour for baking. Then there is the thing that comes after—independence, profession, accountability. There should be one moment when heroes are made, when shoes are stepped into, when destiny is assumed. Neil should have this; he has worked hard for it and is certainly deserving. He should speak with confidence and in a tone that does not allow room for doubt.

"Have you ever used one?" Alli asks again.

Neil's voice cracks. Instead of becoming taller or more powerful in appearance, he simply stays the same size.

"On a doll," he tells her.

Alli slaps the instrument into his waiting hand without a pause and answers, "That's good enough."

It is a ridiculous moment that we should have laughed over when it happened, because this was not the way medicine should be practiced, could be practiced, in a place of such renown and prestige. We had all fought hard to gain our admission into this program, but we did so with the understanding that we would be guided gently by those with far more experience than we. It is impossible that we are standing alone in a stairwell without an attending and no help on the way.

It makes sense for the very first time only when we finally burst into the delivery room to find, not a pregnant mother of premature triplets, but donuts and coffee with balloons floating overhead.

There is a buoyant postmortem of the prank by all who were involved. The attending who had been running rounds demands confirmation that we had been stricken, convinced by his demeanor that he was a force to be reckoned with. We do as we are expected, nodding in complicity that yes, we had been terrified. In this hierarchy of the hospital that is intern, then resident, and then attending, it would be unthinkable to do anything but agree, so the whole fete is declared a success.

We were not alone in being made active participants in such a performance. In the Children's Hospital next door and the old City Hospital a few miles away, horrified interns had watched as diapers smeared with brownie mix were licked by nurses, as urine containers filled with apple juice were unhesitatingly drunk from, and as code bells in various units went off simultaneously. It was the sort of hazing that begets its own propagation as class after class vows to one-up the strange and bizarre scenarios that are played out for them, conspiring each year to make the roles and the scripts at once more shocking and more believable. Only the woman who is to be Neil's and my attending shakes her head and says, "I can't believe they still do this. It was crazy when I was a resident and it's still crazy now."

In the end, though, we were all to be pediatricians, a field within medicine not usually remarked upon for its hard-ass personalities, and the day, unusual though it had been, was brought to a close with some measure of welcome.

"If you're not having fun, then you need to tell me," the head of the unit gathered us up to say. "If you're not having fun, then we're doing something wrong."

Then we pair off with the seasoned interns we will be replacing to hand off patients and the responsibility that goes with them—a ritual that will be repeated every four weeks for the next three years.

That afternoon, at home, my husband Daryl sits at the dining room table with his unfinished thesis assembled in piles of loose scrap paper before him, equations tumbling along the edges of cocktail napkins and on the back of Stop & Shop receipts.

"How was it?" he asks.

I collapse onto the couch slowly and in well-controlled free fall to give the kittens Oryx and Crake enough time to roll lazily out of my way. "It was okay, I think. The people are nice, at least, so that's something."

"What time do you have to be there tomorrow? The same as today?"

"No." I close my eyes as the kittens start to purr and let my head fall back onto the pillows behind me. "From now on, I have to be there even earlier."

On the day that I graduated medical school, I became a doctor, and yet, despite the framed awards I was handed and the green hood that was so ceremoniously draped over my shoulders to hang down my back, I was in no way qualified to practice medicine. I had become very good at taking standardized tests, neatly filling in ovals with my number 2 pencil or clicking my answers on the new computerized exams that were held in rooms that seemed designed to be always exactly the wrong temperature and not at all conducive to performing at your best. Perhaps this was on purpose. There would be nothing about the three years I would spend as a resident that would be comfortable. I would learn to think and act quickly despite hunger and fatigue and being long overdue for a trip to the bathroom. The three years of pediatrics residency that followed were a training period that seemed at times a sort of purgatory, an indentured servitude from which I would never escape. It seemed impossible that the promised transformation—of bumbling intern into practiced attending—could take place in so short a time.

Despite the brutal schedule, we were strongly encouraged to consider ourselves lucky. We did not live in the hospital, as doctors in training used to do, despite spending the majority of our waking hours there. We were, in fact, not permitted to work for more than thirty hours at a stretch. We were required to be given a period of twenty-four hours away from the hospital at least once a week. We could have no fewer than ten hours in between ending one shift and beginning the next. We were, in a word, soft. There were supervising physicians who would raise their eyebrows if complaints were made within their hearing, and the weak, spineless intern who had been up for only just a little bit more than a day would likely then be regaled with a lengthy dissertation on how medicine could only be learned from the bedside, by watching the evolution of an illness from start to finish, admission to discharge, without ever going home. It was the medical equivalent of walking to school three miles in the snow, going uphill both ways.

The strict rules that govern how long airplane pilots can work at a stretch and how long they must be permitted to rest in between—so important is their performance and reaction time—had never been widely applied to medicine before the American College of Graduate Medical Education (ACGME) made the implementation of resident work hour rules necessary for the accreditation of residency programs in 2003. Some of the work evaluating the effect of fatigue on physician performance had actually been done in the very same hospitals where I would train. Residents who had been awake for extended periods were more likely to make errors in diagnosis and in dosing medications. They were slower to respond to stimuli and more likely to crash their cars after finally leaving the hospital to drive home, since being that tired is the physiologic equivalent of being drunk. When New Jersey passed a law in 2004 making it against the law to drive if you have not slept in the past twenty-four hours, residents in programs in that state were advised to remain in the hospital to take a nap before leaving work.

But even sleeping a little on call was not a viable solution to the underlying problem. Chris Landrigan, the author of many hallmark journal articles on this topic, worked closely with residents. In my final year I would be present at a conference in which he told a story about his toothbrush. Chris had been a resident in our program and had been sleeping in a call room in the ICU when he received a page about a patient with serious breathing troubles who needed to be transferred and intubated immediately. He heard about the patient and probably even asked appropriate questions before hanging up the phone and immediately falling back asleep. When the patient arrived on the unit and Chris was nowhere to be found, a colleague came to his call room and shook him awake. The patient was on the unit, he was told, and needed a breathing tube to be placed. Chris woke up and nodded, then stood and walked to the bathroom to brush his teeth. He was suffering from sleep inertia, an inability during that transition from sleep to full wakefulness to appropriately respond no matter how smart or organized or well-meaning you are. It was a feeling I would come to know well—the haze and the grogginess—almost as well as its opposite (lack-of-sleep inertia), during the three years I would spend in the Boston Combined Residency Program (BCRP) in pediatrics.

These three years of training would be divided between the Children's Hospital in Boston, affiliated with the Harvard Medical School, and Boston Medical Center, the Boston University hospital a few miles (but a significant distance) away. Though the majority of other training programs have links to a university, the BCRP is associated with two. Early in the 1990s, the program directors of both the Harvard Children's and Boston University programs took the unprecedented step to combine these into one residency in order to provide their residents with more breadth and depth of training than either institution could offer alone. Experience with the wealth of subspecialty services and technology-driven procedures at Children's would be combined with the "bread-and-butter" pediatrics of Boston Medical Center, where issues surrounding access to care and advocacy for the underserved were the driving forces behind their mission statement: "Exceptional Care Without Exception." The result for the more than one hundred residents serving in all classes at any given time was an unparalleled educational opportunity. Its only drawback was that the multitude of inpatient services needing coverage between the two hospitals (and the Brigham nurseries next door to Children's) meant that residents rarely had the time to appreciate this privilege.

I was halfway through my internship when I realized that there was no way that I would finish. I was unhappy. It's possible I was even depressed, because the symptoms of depression—fatigue, impaired concentration, insomnia and hypersomnia, psychomotor retardation, and recurrent thoughts of death—seemed inescapable while doing this job. Courtesy of the noontime conference lunches and the cafeteria food that was my only option during nights on call, I even had significant weight gain. So I told my program directors that I did not think that I would make it. I needed some time to decompress, to get my head in order, to write down all the things I'd seen and experienced since the first day in the NICU when Alli led us running down the hall.

Admitting that I needed help was hard. Not as hard as continuing residency uninterrupted would have been, as my colleagues can attest to, but difficult still. Sitting with our program director, Bob Vinci, in his small office at Boston Medical Center, I had made what I thought would be interpreted as a rather desperate plea. I would be seen as weak. I would be thought of as lazy. But I was too tired and overwhelmed to really care. Instead, he said to me, "How much time do you need?" And I, in return, asked, "How much time can I have?"

Fred Lovejoy (the Harvard Children's program director) suggested that I should take my time and finish the training in four years instead of three. I appreciated the support he was giving, but I also had a mortgage and student loans to pay. Even with both my husband and I working full-time, we had to be careful each month in order to pay our bills. I knew that this was a project that could easily go bust. It would be necessary to plan carefully how best to minimize the damage, to save face and move on.

In a smaller program my request might have presented problems, but in a mammoth organization such as the BCRP there was a certain amount of wiggle room.

There was still the matter of the call schedule—a complicated grid of day and nighttime work assignments for the dozen or so inpatient services that needed coverage in addition to two ERs. One less body would mean more work for everyone else, so Bob had to think carefully before he answered my question. "What if you work for three four-week blocks at a time and then take four weeks off? Will that be enough?" Four whole weeks to turn off my pager, sleep late, go out to dinner with friends, and (yes) write sounded wonderful. I would finish out my internship, I decided, since I was more depressed by the idea of having it hanging over me than by the need to continue to show up to work every day. Then, at the start of my junior year, I would adopt a modified schedule that would allow me time to write.

As a senior, I went back to working nearly full-time. I would finish residency just sixteen weeks late. Given the real possibility (had I been determined to just soldier on) of spiraling into a breakdown and not finishing at all, it was well worth the delay.

And I wrote a book. I slept in and lost track of my pager and watched more than my share of *Criminal Minds* during the four-week chunks when I was not working, but I wrote some stories as well. I had met many families and had cared for their children during times of incredible strain. There were stories of extraordinary tenderness and devotion, of mothers and fathers keeping watch through the white painted bars of a hospital crib. There were stories of incalculable bravery, of the girl who barely survived the shooting deaths of all of her family by her mentally ill brother and still found the courage to remember how to smile. There were stories of fear and of hope and of all of those emotions that lie in between. But they were in so many ways not mine to share. My stories, in which I am too often petty and spiteful and always so much less than I wish I could be, are the only ones I am really qualified to tell. Those other stories are also here in the pages that follow, but because they have been borrowed, I know that there are bound to be things I have gotten wrong. Also, because all of these families are entitled to privacy, there are many details and names that I have had to change. Still these stories are as true as I knew how to make them, and I can only hope they manage to convey a small fraction of the admiration I have for those parents who are faced with the serious illness of a child.

Now, having finished my training, I still work at Children's. It is the sort of place from which it is difficult to escape. We grow used to the ease with which we can consult a myriad of specialists for that difficult diagnosis, the peace of mind that comes from knowing your patients are being watched by the best nurses even during those times you are called away from the floor, the phlebotomists and IV team and sedation services that are so crucial to patients' needs. But also it has become familiar; its floors have begun to feel (filled as they are with so many friends who are also colleagues) more than just a little like a kind of home.

There is a saying in medicine that if you hear hoofbeats, you should think of horses, not zebras. The message being that, common things being common, it is important to address the more likely diagnoses first. But I had, during my three years of training, seen more than a few zebras. The lesson there, I would like to believe, is that it is always important to adjust your expectations when events do not play out the way you thought that they would. For instance, I had not expected to be sorry to leave residency. But I was. True, I was too drunk on sleep and freedom to notice, but there were still moments when I missed being a part of something so big. And I had not expected, even when enormously pregnant, to ever actually become a mother. But I did, and I quickly realized two things. First, I was even more tired than I was when an intern. And second, I knew absolutely nothing about babies when I was writing this book, before I finally got to take care of my own.

Glorioso

"Whisper," you tell me. "Don't talk any louder."

I am not a good person. I am not remarkably kind. Still, I can follow directions, so I lower my voice so that no one can hear.

"I'm confused."

You don't look at me, but I imagine your eyes as they would be if you were older, if they could open, if time did not stand still. I make them blue and I endow them with wisdom, this pair of irises and lenses. I imagine your eyes as I wish they could be.

"Of course you are," you reply. "Did you think you were special? There have been others before you and it is always the same."

I stand, awkward and uncertain at the foot of the incubator, and pull at the knot of woven string at my waist. The scrubs I am wearing, starched and fresh from the hospital laundry, hang loose and balloon out in all the wrong places. Catching sight of myself in a darkened computer screen or glass partition, it is like seeing a body that has been submerged, has become bloated and irreconcilable with what it once was.

In the summer months of that first year of residency there are still one or two hours of daylight remaining when I leave the neonatal intensive care unit where the smallest and most fragile of our young patients are held. With the memory of the sun warm on my skin, it is possible to believe that my face and my body had one day been beautiful, although they never were. It is possible to breathe slowly, first in and then out, and to measure these breaths by the heartbeats in between. It is possible, standing on the tile squares of stained linoleum and draped in cheap blue cloth of the sort we used to cut dolls from, to remember a self that was pretty if not beautiful, generous if not kind, and ordinary above all. It was a life assembled from nothing remarkable, that was no more extraordinary than puddles splashing under sandaled feet or a forgiving breeze wending along the backs of sweaty knees, but it had been mine entirely and even now—diminished though I had become, squeezed though I was into the handful of minutes that framed each work day—I still had sun. Facing the incubator where my very first patient lies naked beneath the bare electric coils that are meant to warm him, I begin to suspect that it is the ordinary things that are the most precious, and it is with a feeling of dread that I realize it will be these I am least able to bestow.

"So I am not any different."

You have had other doctors. Already in your lifetime there have been three sets of interns standing where I am, peering in through the plastic walls that divide us, lifting the edge of the quilted coverings that, like oversized tea cozies, help to block out the light.

"Did you want to be different?" you ask me, and I am embarrassed, for I did shyly but desperately wish that I could be.

I would not be the most clever—that much I knew for certain even this early on. I would not be the most hardworking, the most confident or sincere. So I did not hope to be better than those doctors who stood there before me, their white coats as fresh and unstained as the one I had been handed only several days before, but neither did I want to be entirely faceless. If different was the most that I could hope for, then to be anything less was to have failed.

Instead, I fumble, unable to put a voice to this muted desperation even within the confines of my own skull: "I don't know. I can't imagine it matters."

I rest the heel of one silk shoe on the toe of the other. They are shoes that I know look altogether too much like slippers to be practical. The silver, orange, and blue threads of embroidery would fray over the course of a few short weeks and the flat rubber soles would leave my feet aching at the end of each day. Still I persisted and wore them anyway for protection, believing they would act as a talisman, because it would be unthinkable that someone wearing such precious shoes could be anything short of cheerful, could be scuffing the floors of hallways along which children might actually die.

"Not to me, you mean."

"Not to you."

You are sixty-eight days old and still nearly two months premature, born unforgivably soon at twenty-four weeks and some change. You have been given a name, Connor, after a cousin on your father's side who was killed by shrapnel from a roadside bomb in Anbar only days after arriving in Iraq. You have been christened by a Catholic priest who rolled back his shirt cuffs to reveal slender, feminine wrists and who reached in through two opened portals on one side of your cocoon to sprinkle you with water and press holy oil on the crown of your tiny head. You have been loved, cruelly and completely, and you have not been let go.

"How could it matter?" you ask. "I don't actually exist."

"Exactly."

Connor becomes mine on the very first morning of my training, by which time I have read all about him, have scoured his chart and his vitals, the lists of medications and procedures, the reports from the ultrasounds that show the blood in his brain. I have counted the number of times that he almost died, including the six occasions his doctors had to push epinephrine and the week that (in order to ward off further disaster) the defibrillator was permanently parked next to his bed. I know that his parents are named Missy and Charles, although I have never met them. They were young; they were childless. So when they were presented with needles and catheters and tubing and scalpels, they did not ever say no.

When Missy's water broke at the end of her twenty-third week, they said, "Yes. We want everything," and that is precisely what they got. It was natural, this desire, to nurture and protect. Everything, as if they were ordering from a dessert menu or choosing a vacation with all the possible perks. But everything, when you go to a restaurant or a travel agent, has a logical limit to what it might mean. In the hospital, for a child, everything changes, every day it becomes different, and the line is pushed further and further until at some point the pain that is inflicted outweighs all the possible good. It is these times when everything is too much.

In the weeks before I came onto the service, they had tried to feed him, running the tiniest volume of formula down a tube that went in through Connor's nose to end in his stomach. The calories this trickle provided were negligible, were enough really only to feed the lining of his gut. It was a reminder to these cells of the job they would someday be called on to perform if all else went better than could possibly be hoped. It was at that point that his abdomen expanded, little by little, darkening toward blackness as the distension increased. It was a sign that the inside surface of his intestines, unable to muster enough blood flow to sustain itself during the challenging task of absorbing nutrients, had started to die.

At that point the surgeon had come to tell Missy and Charles that Connor's abdomen was filled with dead bowel, but that he had no way of knowing the extent of the damage that had been done. If Connor had been stable, if his blood pressure was not bottoming out and if it was only the necrotizing enterocolitis that he was faced with, then the next step would have been surgery, would have been to open him up and run the length of his bowel between gloved fingertips to determine the parts that should be resected and the bits that could be saved.

"If he were your child," Missy and Charles had asked the surgeon. "If he were yours, then what would you do?"

And the middle-aged father of three had looked at them each both in turn in their eyes and said to them honestly, "I would let him go."

But Missy had shaken her head. Missy, whose last pregnancy had ended at twenty weeks and who so keenly mourned the loss of a child she never saw, blinked quickly to clear the wetness from her eyes, and she shook her head.

Charles spoke for the both of them when he said, "We want everything done."

The surgeon had not cut Connor open, had not exposed the loops of healthy pink and glistening intestine and the gray lifeless tissue that needed to be thrown away. It was there he drew the line. With the preemie's pulses barely palpable and his heart rate winding down, the surgeon knew the operation would have killed him before they had even started the work that needed to be done. This is why, when I arrive, Connor has a strawlike drain on each side of his abdomen to let fluid and pus and bacteria flow out. This had not fixed the problem, but it was hoped this stopgap measure might prevent the pressure inside his abdomen from continuing to rise. It had been done the way you might patch a crack in the wall of a house that is rotting from inside out, all the while knowing that the chandeliers and banisters might fall down around you before the more permanent repairs are made.

I lay two fingers on either side of the clear dressing that holds both drains in place and press as gently as I can. His belly is still too big for his tiny body. I leave one hand resting against him. Tapping the knuckles of my left hand lightly with my right is like batting at a balloon, and I can hear the mellow tympany of the gas that is inside.

His gut is still not moving properly then, which is not surprising given the purulent fluid that his abdomen continues to drain. I press again, upward and underneath his ribs. From out of the corner of one eye, I almost believe that I see him wincing, pursing the lips of a mouth that is not covered in tape and that might be moved to either smile or frown.

"I'm sorry," I tell Connor, though in reality he does not stir.

"Everyone says that." I imagine him shrugging, imagine him turning away. He should have a window to look out into the distance, in contemplation, even just for effect. He should have so many things that will never be his, but he should have a window at least to begin. Inside his shroud, Connor's shoulders rattle from side to side, his birdlike ribs tremble, his hips remain relatively still. There is an art to adjusting the settings on this ventilator, since it does not measure the volume of each breath but rather the frequency with which each miniscule whiff of fresh air is pulsed into the tube that connects with Connor's lungs, and this is the result, a perverse sort of dance to a record that keeps playing over and over and does not ever stop. It is the reason I lose myself at times in this fanciful dialogue, because there are too many things that are not said out loud.

"Does it hurt?" I ask, pressing deeper, probing for the edge of a liver but meeting only resistance from all the swelling inside.

"I don't know."

It must hurt—every day, every minute.

"I wouldn't know the difference."

This is a blessing, in a way, but realizing this only makes me feel worse.

"We should be able to do better," I think, even though I cannot really picture what better would mean.

"I'm here," he says to me, even though he is sleeping, is so sedated that not even his eyelids flicker when he is touched. "Isn't that enough?"

His parents, if asked this, would say that it is. Before Connor was born, they blushed modestly when they were congratulated that they were expecting a child, a son. "As long as he's healthy," they said, it did not matter if he had Charles's chin, which was bulbous and slightly askew, or Missy's asthma. And when he was half dead and on multiple infusions just to keep his heart beating, they had leaned close, counted ten fingers and ten toes, and decided that was enough. Even after his nose blackened from lack of blood flow and two of those fingers fell off, they counted the fingers that were remaining; they gingerly reached in to stroke the slick sole of one purple foot. "He doesn't have to be beautiful," they told each other, believing that it was true.

They were in the process of rewriting their lives. They were doing what all other good parents must, whittling down the seemingly endless possibilities and then taking stock of what they had left. They would have to be careful with pictures, because of that nose, would have to find an angle where the shadows made it look all right. There would not be piano lessons, but a drum set might be fun even though it would keep up the neighbors. And even if he wasn't any good at baseball or soccer, it didn't mean that he couldn't play. He would get the same cheap plastic trophy at the end of the season anyway. Aren't all children imperfect somehow? Missy and Charles must have reasoned; don't they all, eventually, for a time, disappoint? They cry unexpectedly, for no reason, in the middle of a shopping mall or a restaurant lobby. They make scenes; they embarrass, until people begin to look on in disapproval. Children lie, brazenly and without an echo of guilt, about how the gold-leafed saucer came to be broken, blaming the wind or the dog, conjuring earthquakes or stealthy ninja-like warriors, painting themselves as champions because it is a miracle, really, that there was no more damage than only a saucer; it is a miracle the house is still standing after all it endured.

Still, Connor was broken in ways that they couldn't see. Missy and Charles would be called on to forgive more than they could conceive.

"No," I whisper sadly. "This is not nearly enough. It doesn't even come close."

I do not want Connor to die, but neither do I, blithely and at unlimited cost, want him to live. It is not merely a matter of this day or the next one, or even of each of the long string of weeks that would all together bring Connor to the age he was meant to be when he was born. It is not merely a matter of keeping him breathing, since he is not doing that, since there is a machine that is doing that for him, the jet beating each tiny puff of air in toward his lungs, pushing oxygen in and letting the carbon dioxide diffuse out. If it were only these things, neatly packaged and enveloped in space and time, then I would shrug as Missy and Charles do and say fine, knowing it will be over someday. But it will never be over, not really, not in the way that they think.

The road that Connor is traveling does not end at a wrought iron gate trailing with ivy on the other side of which is a secret garden and the healthy child they had dreamed they would have. If he lives, if he manages somehow to triple and then quadruple his mass to reach the minimum weight that is required for discharge, then this will be only the first step in a long journey that will last the rest of his life. He will return to the hospital, sometimes weekly, for visits with each of his many doctors. There will be a neurologist to manage the seizures that the bleeding into his brain will likely cause. An ophthalmologist will check regularly on the tiny hemorrhages at the back of his eyes and prescribe thick, cartoonish glasses if he is able to see at all. The gastroenterologists and nutritionists will help to monitor his G-tube, a small portal through the skin of his abdomen and into his stomach, since he will choke on any food or liquid that is placed in his mouth. The pulmonologist will prescribe inhalers to protect his airways against the inflammation triggered every day when he breathes his own saliva down into his lungs. And the orthopedists will prescribe braces for his ankles and legs to keep them from stiffening and contracting during the long hours he will spend in his wheelchair because he lacks the strength and coordination to stand.

These are the things Missy and Charles should learn to anticipate so that it becomes possible—just possible—that Connor will exceed expectations instead of the other way round.

"I won't remember any of this," I imagine him saying. "Why does it make you upset?"

"It feels like torture," I tell him. "Every day, with every procedure, we move closer to cruelty. We should be here to protect you."

I am going too far and I know it, but Connor's body is shaking. He had failed the traditional ventilators, had developed a huge pocket of air in his left lung that would fill more with each breath and compress the comparatively healthy lung tissue beside it. He could not breathe on his own, but neither could he tolerate breaths the way they should be delivered, all at once and then out again, because that bleb was expanding and would eventually burst, popping the way a birthday balloon does when the party is ended and the guests have dispersed, violently shredding beyond all hopes of repair.

"Are you sure that that's what this is, that torture is the right word?"

I shake my head as I crouch lower beside him, peeking beneath the papery blankets that are decorated with slightly drugged-looking dogs wearing blue sailor's caps. There is nothing that I am sure of and every day edges become blurrier; the faces of nurses from different shifts melt into one another and names remain elusive, ID badges somehow conspiring to always flip and turn backward, so they cannot be read. This sense that I will always and forever be a stranger here only reinforces the feeling of transience, a feeling that is not allayed even by the reliable and resolute passage of time.

"I think one of my patients is going to die."

The one weekend of that month that I am not working, my parents deliver a carload of our wedding gifts to us from Buffalo. They climb the several flights up to our rented apartment and deposit the plunder—the flatware, the silver candlesticks, the coffee bean grinder—in the front hall. Oryx and Crake hide beneath our bed and only reluctantly allow Daryl to pick them up. My mother and father sit on our newly purchased blue couch, sipping water from tumblers, inspecting this hastily slapped-together home that we've made.

Hanging on the walls are our various treasures: a print of the White Mountains given to us by the couple who—decades ago—had introduced my parents; another print of my college in Oxford that Daryl had bought the previous year when he was still living abroad and I was finishing medical school; a batik purchased in Swaziland with my friend Ellen, who I visited during the year she was teaching for the Peace Corps in Mozambique; a circular Mayan calendar of carved stone from our honeymoon in Belize. These were the most adult-looking things that we owned, so we had arranged them as carefully as we had the furniture in this first place that we lived in, just the two of us, hoping that the things themselves were enough to give a lasting impression to whoever might come to visit that we were doing all right.

We talk about Connor that night at dinner, stopping first in the Market below the MacLean Meats placard that had once hung over my great-grandfather's stalls and then finding our way up the stairs to Durgin Park, where, my mother promised, the waitresses would be wonderfully impatient and rude, just as they always had been, just as she remembered from when she was a girl. We talk about Connor and I offer his possible death up to my family almost as if I am boasting.

I say, "I think one of my patients is going to die," but what I mean is, "I am important enough to be privy to the death of a child; I am important enough to bear witness to events that you never will."

"That's awful," my mother replies.

"It might be more awful if he were to live. His parents push way too hard."

"He's their son."

"If he lives, if he survives, they have no idea of what they might get in the end. They think he'll be normal. He'll never be that."

"What's normal?"

"They think that he'll walk, play in the yard, go to school. They think he'll know who they are. He might not even know that."

My mother adjusts the napkin laid across her lap.

"Maybe that won't matter to them. There are people who do it. The couple at dad's church, their daughter's thirteen, the one in the wheelchair, and they have other children, but they handle it beautifully."

"Then they are the exception."

"What do you think you should do differently?"

I do not need to think before I give my answer, because this is the thing that consumes my thoughts yet is never discussed during the hours when I am at the hospital and there are medications that are added and decisions that are made. I keep hoping I am wrong about the way things will play out, the brightest possible future that I see for Connor, and all the suffering and disappointment it will contain. I want to believe that the things we are doing to him—the infusions of sedatives, the daily needle sticks to draw blood—are being done for good purpose. I want to be told that the end will indeed justify even the most agonizing means, but I am afraid to ask. Instead, I say nothing, filled with too much doubt as to what the verdict will be.

"I think we should say no," I tell my parents, "when a child has endured so much and the options aren't good ones. We should say to the families, this is where it ends. We don't seem to do that and there always seems to be more. If he dies, if we finally come to a point where to go on would be cruelty, we shouldn't have to ask his parents for permission to stop. We should decide that; it should be our fault. It shouldn't be theirs. It's too much power; it's too much responsibility, too much potential for guilt. We should take whatever blame there is that needs to be given. We should give them that one small thing at least."

My mother nods thoughtfully and then asks, "And what if he lives?"

This time I pause, but just for a moment.

"Then they need to know what kind of child they might have to care for, who it is they will be called on to love."

Early on, I keep my distance; after the first day when I approach them for introductions, I stay back. The time that Missy and Charles spend with Connor at the side of the incubator should, I reason to myself, have privacy enough for their grieving, for mourning the loss of so much, even if these losses have stopped short of his actual life. My contact with Connor is limited, in any case, by his nurses, and Margaret, the senior RN who cares for him during the day, is particularly fierce. It is the nature of NICU nurses to be territorial and protective; they control access to the infants in much the same way that a wild animal might lie in wait at the entrance to her den. These nurses, incredible in their skill and devotion, vary in their tolerance of intruders into their world. Here, still, I am an intruder whose inexperienced hands could dislodge catheters and chest tubes even during the most cursory of physical exams. The orders I write for diagnostic imaging or a feed advance are subject to nursing approval, so from the beginning I am made aware of where the real power lies. At times, just to approach an isolette is to risk being on the receiving end of an emphatic vocal reproach. I find myself walking on tiptoe, as if a predator is lurking ever near.

In the late afternoon of one of my weekend calls, Missy and Charles blow kisses at Connor as they turn to leave. After they are gone, I overhear Margaret and the other nurses talking.

"They don't have any idea," they say with both pity and a subtle note of fault, and I realize then that this is hard for them as well.

There was another boy, just as desperately young as Connor, just as sick, and he had died after a hundred days under their care just before Connor was born.

"Do you ever say anything to them?" I ask.

Margaret smiles at me for the first and perhaps only time: "That's not our place."

And I nod solemnly because I know that she is telling me that it is mine.

Still the relationship that Missy and Charles have with Connor's nurses is not one I can hope to achieve. I will be permitted to look on during a brief window of time, to witness the near misses and the moments of small success, remaining mostly anonymous, only to recede into the background again. His nurses, not his doctors, are their daily contacts. It is they who take the late-night phone calls from Missy or Charles, not because his doctors are not willing to take the time, but because it is the nurses' familiar voices his parents want to hear.

So we have spoken only briefly and about things of little consequence. I have told Missy that Connor's epinephrine infusion has been turned up or down or been shut off completely. I have asked her how she's doing, to which she answers, "Fine," always with the same inflection and scripted cheer. I have heard the genuine and undiluted joy in Missy's voice when she tells me how she helped Margaret to bathe him, wiping gently with a cloth the narrow swaths of skin that are not covered over by tape or Tegaderm. I have been told by Charles in a tone of such unbridled optimism that Connor looks so much better, has grown so big, that I had turned, almost expecting a miraculous transformation, but finding instead that he still is not much longer than one of my hands.

Several days later there is a family meeting, a scheduled opportunity for the attending physician and the fellow to speak at once with both Missy and Charles about the progress that has been made. Connor is still alive. The drains in his abdomen are there, untouched, because the surgeons (with a small measure of necessary restraint) are still unwilling to do anything more. All of the calories that he is given are entering through a vein, through a long IV line that has been threaded (when all other access points were lost) through a small vessel in his scalp and down his neck to end in one of the larger vessels just above his heart. The medications that have been used to maintain his blood pressure have been weaned and one of them has been shut off.

"He's made some excellent steps forward," Michelle, the fellow, tells Connor's parents when she has finished this update.

"I know," Charles says. "We've been really happy that he's been doing so well. His belly's not so swollen. He doesn't seem to be in as much pain."

Michelle had chosen her words carefully; she had been clear and she had even at times been blunt, yet it seems that she had not actually been heard. There is barely a pause before the attending leans forward because she sees exactly what is happening. She has seen it too many times before. So she says without waiting, "He's on quite a lot of fentanyl to keep him from being agitated, to keep him from feeling some of the pain."

In that moment, she becomes my hero. She could have stayed silent, could have left the feeling of accomplishment afloat in the air, unsullied and complete. But that would have been lying just the same as if she had chosen to speak a falsehood to Charles's face.

"All of the things that we've discussed up until now have been true. Connor's done much better than we had expected he could when we last sat down. He's made some very real steps. But there are things that you still need to be very aware of—some of them we've talked about before. The bleeding in his brain—it doesn't look like there's been any more of it, but the damage is still there. We don't know if that's the reason he's had such trouble keeping his blood pressure up on his own. We don't know what sort of deficits he'll have in the long run because of it."

Missy and Charles give the appearance that they are listening and I begin to have hope that there is a way to care for these infants that is both tenacious and true, both heroic and humane.

"There's also some very real damage to his lungs from his prematurity, and he's on the jet, the specialized ventilator we've gone over before, meaning he's very far away from breathing on his own. We also don't know what's going on in his belly. We don't know how much of the bowel in there will be functional, how much of it has already died. It's likely that he'll need surgery, not now, because he's still not stable, but at some point, to take that dead gut out. How he'll do afterward, how that will affect how well he's able to grow, will depend on how much is left."

It is a sobering speech. It has been necessary but somehow does not seem the right place to end.

Then the attending says, "Still, he's hanging in there. He's a strong little boy."

Just as quickly as they were assumed, the looks of studious attentiveness vanish. Missy absently rubs at the tattoo on her right arm, a small rose that curls perfectly just below her deltoid and that must have been placed after she lost all the extra weight the stretch marks just beside it tell me she once had.

"Thanks so much," Charles says. "We couldn't be more thrilled with how he's doing."

I am upset by the blithe way in which Missy and Charles seem to dismiss these final warnings, and I leave the meeting feeling somewhat defeated. But, after hearing the bladelike edge in my attending's voice, I find that I am no longer afraid that it would be overstepping to speak similarly, to acknowledge that nothing is certain, that everything could still be lost.

The next time Missy visits, Charles is with her. They sit beside Connor in two matching rocking chairs, chatting with each other, looking in at their son with contented smiles on their faces. I can tell from the way that they are turned in, facing each other, that they are not looking for company, but I approach them anyway because I ambitiously think that it is possible that I was mistaken, that they have understood certain things that I know to be important, but I want to find out for sure.

"You've had a couple of days now to think over the things that were discussed at the meeting. Do you have any questions that didn't get covered?"

Missy and Charles share a look between the two of them and they shrug dismissively.

She says, "We know that he's still got some stuff going on, but when will we have a better idea of when he can come home?"

I feel my chest go quiet inside me, feel my heart miss a beat. My voice is harsher than usual and this is on purpose. I want them to listen to what I have to say.

"Connor will have to be able to do certain things before he's ready to go, and the same list of things applies to any infant here. He'll need to be able to maintain his own body temperature. He's not doing that. The isolette is doing it for him and his skin is too thin now to keep in the heat. He needs to gain weight, and while he is doing that, we're still not feeding him through his gut. He needs to breathe on his own; right now the ventilator is doing that for him. He needs to maintain a normal blood pressure without all of the medications that he's on. At the very least, he'll be here until his due date, which is still more than a month away, but he's a very sick little boy. There are many things that need to go exactly right for him between now and then in order for him to survive."

Charles is still rocking thoughtfully in his chair.

"We have a great backyard where Missy grows roses," he tells me. "We can barbecue there and play soccer. I can't wait until he's big enough so I can grill him his first steak."

It occurs to me first that he must be kidding. I take a deep breath and then I try again.

"If Connor lives, if he survives, he may never walk. He may not be able to swallow; he may not be able to chew. So even if he has enough bowel left to keep him growing, it doesn't mean he'll eat normally. Children with the sort of problems that Connor has often have to have a special tube placed between the outside of their belly and their stomach inside. They don't eat through their mouths."

They are asking so much every day from Connor, and this is what I am asking in return—that they consider what they might get when all this is over, and to consider that when it is over for us, for them it has only just begun. Missy and Charles sit in front of me. They do not ask questions. Later when they get up to leave, Charles glares at me down the hall while I am talking with Michelle, the fellow who is with me on call.

"You did the right thing, telling them what you did. They need to hear it, probably much more than they have."

This is not the first time Michelle has been there to give encouragement and it will not be the last. Just over three years later, it will be her eyes calmly meeting my own from above her surgical mask while on the other side of a sterile blue drape the obstetricians splash my belly with Betadine to prep for an emergent cesarean. It will be her voice that tells me for the first time that my daughter—who I have not yet seen—is beautiful and that everything is fine. We will share a look that contains within it all the more joy because we both know it might not have been that way.

Standing beside her in the NICU, I say, "I just wonder what happens when he goes home and stops being a baby, when he gets big enough that they start to notice that he's not doing the things that other children all do. I've seen so many other couples bringing their kids in to see the neurologist or their GI doctor, and they are almost all of them divorced and left with this broken kid, this full-time job of caring for a child they both wanted to save but couldn't bear to live with afterward. I think, if they weren't told—when things were being decided—how it could turn out, I think then that's our fault, that divorce. They need to take seriously the things they are choosing."

Michelle had hugged me, saying only, "You'll be all right," because she knew it was what I most needed to hear.

When I am done with the four weeks of this first rotation, I sign out my patients to the intern who will take my place. Connor, one month older than when I met him, appears essentially unchanged. Several of the less premature infants have graduated to the subacute unit down the hall and one of them (I heard) has even been sent home. Still the rows of isolettes in the area in which I worked for so many hours remain full, with new newborns taking the place of all the old. The transfer of information to my replacement takes over an hour.

At home that evening, I sigh to signal to my husband that he should ask what is wrong.

"What happened?" Daryl asks me.

"Nothing." I am giving him an answer, but he doesn't realize it.

"Then what's the problem?" Daryl says with exasperation and shoots me a look that tells me to stop being cryptic.

So I answer, "Nothing got better during these last weeks in the NICU. No one was really fixed."

"So what?"

I pause and consider what is really bothering me.

We had fought several nights before and I had cried at how different it all was from what I had expected, how I was more tired than I had ever thought I could be. He pointedly reminded me that I had chosen this—this program and this city—and he had followed, as if my complicity should erase all possibility of unhappiness, or at the very least, that I should keep it to myself. Only weeks earlier, such bluntness would have destroyed me, but I had learned from Connor that it is possible to write both sides of a conversation, so I told Daryl (with a measure of calm I did not exactly feel but had already learned to outwardly embody) the words that would make me feel better and waited impatiently until he repeated exactly the things I had just told him to say.

Now, trying again to find the right tone, I tell him, "This shouldn't just be all that there is. I'll never know what worked and what didn't. I'll never get to see how things will turn out."

Daryl does not respond, and this time I do not supply any lines for him because I cannot think so soon after leaving Connor and the others what I would want for him to say. Even months later, I remain unsure.

"How are you doing?" I would like to be able to ask Connor. I would like for there to be an answer, a real one, but instead I imagine what his response might be.

"I'm here," he tells me. His eyelashes are darker. There is the faintest suggestion of hair on his head. "I hope that's enough."

I close my eyes and lie back on a narrow bed in the on-call suite. I have no room for promises, but I do still have room for something else.

"I hope so, too."

Sugar Call

"We're not leaving until we speak to the neurology attending."

They do not have classes and seminars on how to tell a family good news, most likely because it is a task that is meant to be simple. In contrast, there are professionally shot videos on bereavement, on how to relate the details of a death. All people involved, the physician and family, should be sitting down. The news should be delivered at eye level by someone who has taken the time to be still, not by some white-coated stranger who is anxiously shifting his or her weight from the left foot to the right, communicating by this unrest that they are ready to flee. There should be quiet. There should be time to reflect. A nurse or other staff member who cared for the deceased should be left with the family while the physician steps away to sign orders, to check in on the other patients still in his or her care. The family should not be left alone and the presence of the nurse is thought to serve as a physical connection to the dead child. After a brief time has passed, the physician is meant to return, to again sit and this time answer questions, having allowed the family some minutes to recover from the initial shock of the loss.

People have studied this. Dissertations have been written. There are entire courses on how to relate a death or a fatal diagnosis or a crippling loss of a limb. Although it is a skill that hopefully will not have to be called upon frequently, the giving of bad news should be done delicately and with some competence at least.

There is no equivalent training on how to impart information at a positive outcome, to confer onto parents the absence of distress. Perhaps this is because in the wake of all of the wrenching sorrow that swirls around us, it is assumed that good news should be relatively easy to give. Unfortunately, nothing in medicine is ever so pure. There is no diagnosis that does not leave with it some small measure of doubt. And the problem is that sometimes bad news, although it is awful, is preferable to an unknown against which you cannot prepare.

The child I am meant to send home today is a seven-year-old boy. He has autism. He has very significant developmental delay. He does not speak, does not interact, does not feed or clothe himself, and he is in the hospital because he has had a seizure and a fever of 101°F. He has had an MRI that shows no structural abnormalities. There is no tumor. There is no mass. There is nothing there to explain the seizure, but then there is nothing there to indicate that he will ever seize again. This is the good news; the neurologists and neuroradiologists have analyzed this boy's case and they have nothing more to say. He is on the General Pediatrics Service and I am meant to walk into his room and tell his parents that his MRI is normal and that they are free to go. It should be simple. It should be painless. And yet I am suddenly faced with a set of angry parents who send me out of the room with the echo of their raised voices still buzzing in my ears.

It is my second month as an intern, and is my first call with Rishi. He is the senior resident supervising for the weekend. When I find him, he asks how things have gone. I am still somewhat bewildered by the attack.

"They demanded to see the neurology attending."

He laughs.

"Did you tell them that it's six o'clock on a Sunday night?"

"I told them that I didn't believe it would be possible."

Rishi tilts his head a bit to one side to indicate his continued amusement. There are hints of what someday may be wrinkles at the corners of his dark eyes as he smiles.

"That was very diplomatic."

I am not sure if this is a compliment or if he is, gently at least and without any malice, making fun.

"They weren't impressed."

"What was the problem?" he asks, though I strongly suspect that he already knows.

I shrug: "I thought that when the neurology team rounded this morning the plan was to get the MRI, and if it was normal, then he would go home."

Rishi purses his brown lips in mock concentration: "That is correct."

"Everyone was there and it was agreed upon. His parents understood."

"That was my impression, too."

"Now they are saying they want to know the reason for the seizure."

"And what did you say?"

"I told them that young children sometimes seize, and that when it's associated with a fever, they are often not even admitted to the hospital."

Rishi leans back and props one leg up on the chair across from where he sits. The thin blue fabric of his scrubs lifts at the ankle to reveal a small hole in the somewhat yellowed sock.

"Do you think this was a simple febrile seizure?"

I pause to hurriedly review my memories of the lecture we had been given earlier in the week, then, "Technically, he's too old."

"Hence the MRI." He waves a hand in the air as if he is willing me to move forward to the next step.

"Yes."

"And his parents are upset because they were told by someone that he is too old for this to just be called a simple febrile seizure."

I lean forward and rest an elbow on the Formica table that stands between us upon which are littered the remains of the day's paperwork, a bag of quickly hardening bagels, and a plastic knife coated with a skin of cream cheese and crumbs.

"They seem to be."

"What did you say then?"

I look up and at the same time exhale in an expression that I hope admits defeat and also garners enough sympathy that I will not be sent in there again.

"I didn't know what to say, and whatever it was that they wanted to hear, they didn't want to hear it from me."

"I can talk to them," he says easily as if it is nothing.

Rishi pulls his leg down in preparation to rise but pauses again.

"What could you have said now that you've had a chance to think it over?"

I look at him helplessly.

"I just don't know."

"Why don't older children have seizures when they are febrile?"

"Because their brains have become much more developed. Their seizure threshold is higher."

"So what could you have told his parents?"

The boy had been unaware of the fight. He had lain in his hospital bed as he would lie in the bed waiting for him at home. He blinks to bright light but does not turn to look for a source. He swallows baby food that is spooned into his mouth but does not open until his lips are gently prodded apart. His mother clucks to him during meals as she had done when he was six months old and just beginning to take solids. The bibs he wears have grown larger, but the ritual is the same.

I am silent.

"What could you have told them?" Rishi asks, softer this time.

"That his brain never really grew up."

In any given day I make a thousand tiny decisions. I calculate drug dosages for a given patient's weight and decide to round up or down. I consider the various side effects and choose Tylenol instead of Motrin. I write for IV fluids with this much potassium to run at such and such a rate. In the beginning, each of these decisions was something to agonize over. I paused over decimal points and the difference between 191 milligrams of ibuprofen and an even 200. I vacillated; I dwelled, unnecessarily and painfully stopping to repeat the simplest multiplications and to recheck the guidelines on the pharmacy web page. It did not make for the greatest efficiency and I slept little if at all the nights that I took call.

The first of these nights I spent in the hospital after leaving the NICU was with Steffie, one of the other residents in Rishi's class.

"Sleeping on call is just not a good idea," she had told me. "You don't know enough yet to know when it is safe and when it is not, so it's better just to be awake and ready."

She had wisps of fine blonde hair framing her face and a mild German accent that made her statements seem all the more convincing. In any case, I knew that she was usually right. Still I needed more than just the passage of time to teach me when it was safe to walk away from a room, to make me believe that if I were called back in an emergency I would know what to do. What I needed most of all was an infusion of confidence, given to me the way we might deliver an antibiotic through an IV. I did not walk away from my overnights with Rishi with quite the same swagger with which he carried himself, but I at least learned not to tiptoe, and that was a start.

"They sent me over to keep a closer eye on you," Rishi would say to me with a wink a month later when I was at the City Hospital and he stopped by to pick up some papers he had to fill out.

It was significant that I did not stop to doubt myself before I laughed. I had learned in just the space of a few short months that we did not come to this phase of our training prepared to do the job that would ultimately be expected of us when we were done. We did not have the knowledge or—at times even more importantly—the finesse to provide reassurance while deflecting the frustrations and the doubts that are manufactured by the stress of seeing a child with sensors across the chest and an IV in an arm or foot. In discharging the boy who had the seizure, Rishi had rescued me. That act of heroism—no more than a few minutes' inconvenience for him but nothing short of miraculous in my eyes—had taught me another thing: that in this process of becoming that grander person, the one with answers to every question and quiet placation for every assault, we are not alone.

The main difficulty in answering questions effortlessly lay not just in the fund of knowledge, factoids that could be easily called up on a computer and presented as evidence during morning rounds. Book learning was quickly reduced to practicalities. I knew, for example, that the IV fluid rates I chose by rote represented actual daily electrolyte requirements, but did not waste time contemplating this fact. I knew that our hospital's approach to treating febrile infants, the blood and urine and cerebrospinal fluid cultures and the forty-eight hours of antibiotic coverage we gave to those under three months of age, was based on a study that had been done in our own ER, but it would take me another two years to read the article for myself. I began to order lab work more quickly, but less reflexively, and with some appreciation of what I expected each test to show.

The main difficulty in answering questions came in realizing that patients and their parents don't obey the same rules of chapter headings and indexed references that structured our education. They ask questions for the sake of asking them, to feel involved, much as children do when they are three or four. And while this sort of ritual has its own distinct value, there are times when a mother might as well be asking why the sky is not indigo and a father might inquire why people do not walk upside down.

"Isn't there some other test that you can do?"

There are five children in the room when Andre's mother poses this question to me, and only one of them is my patient. His four younger siblings are slapping each other and then ducking noisily away from retaliation in the small square of open space situated between the television and Andre's bed. Andre ignores them as he is ignoring his mother's unnecessarily urgent query, the gravity of the situation no doubt amplified by the inconvenience associated with having to visit her eldest child in the hospital without having anyone to watch her three daughters and her other son.

Andre had come in for evaluation of abdominal pain. In the course of his emergency room examination, his stool test was positive for blood. Upon further inquiry by the resident who did his initial workup, Andre admitted that sometimes his feces were bright red. Because of this finding and because Andre had persisted in his claim that the pain he was having was excruciating, he had been admitted for observation. I was not familiar with the particulars of his case, as he was cared for more directly by another intern on my team. I did know, however, that his condition was not thought serious and that it was generally agreed upon that after another day's observation he would likely be discharged home.

"We've done bloodwork that shows that his hematocrit is stable, a measure of red blood cells that tells us that his bleeding can't be very severe."

Andre's mother is not satisfied. Before she responds, she stoops and uses one thick arm to bat away a small hand that is pulling at his sister's braids.

Then, "But where's the bleeding coming from?"

"Likely from somewhere lower down in his GI tract based on the color of his stool."

"But how do you know? Isn't there some way to look?"

I tell her, "That's a great question," because it is.

"There's a procedure we call a colonoscopy," I continue. "It is the same test that older people have done routinely to check the colon for signs of cancer, but basically it's just a way to take a look at the inside of the bowel wall. We use a very small camera that's passed through the GI tract starting from below."

"Why hasn't Andre had that done?"

"Every procedure has some risk involved," I try to explain. "And we would need to be convinced that doing the colonoscopy would actually be useful and give us enough information to make that risk worthwhile. But Andre's bleeding seems to have stopped, and common things being common, he likely had some constipation that caused just a little bit of tearing around his rectum when he passed hard stools. Those are tears that should heal nicely on their own. He shouldn't be exposed to the risks of sedation and anesthesia if he is already getting better."

She considers this for a moment with every appearance of a woman who is slowly but appropriately processing the information she has been given. I expect her to nod at any moment and to take the other children home. She will gather them up and stop the girls from biting their brother in retaliation for the hair tugging and then she will thank me for carefully explaining our reasons for treating Andre's case in the way we have with careful observation and pain control. She will agree that all has been handled properly and is as it should be.

Instead, she awkwardly clutches a handful of denim shirt with fingers tipped in azure press-on nails and pulls at the shoulder strap of her brassiere to readjust one enormous breast.

"I want the camera thing."

* * *

I leave Andre's room with a sense of disquiet that I can't quite place. I had tried to be firm in my assessment that a colonoscopy would not be needed and as such would not be done. To be anything less than definitive is to invite more confusion than I already had created, to lay the groundwork for discord and to have questions raised later that one of my colleagues would have to face. This is why I had been unsuccessful the evening I had tried to pacify the parents of the boy with the seizure—because they had been told something that made them believe he should not be let go. It is not that I doubt whether everything I told Andre's mother is correct, although as usual I do. It is also not that I regret slightly having been so forthcoming about what sorts of tests are sometimes done, although I do. But rather the uneasiness that is weighing on me as I leave Andre behind for a time is like a dense and murky fog that I cannot see clearly through. What I have suddenly become not entirely sure of is that we are treating Andre with as much care and sensitivity as we would if he were white.

Rishi and I stop in to check on a boy from New Hampshire. Brandon is a soccer player who will enter his sophomore year at Groton or Exeter or Andover or Choate in the fall. From the tasteful brooch on his mother's cashmere sweater, I guess that their front yard is neatly partitioned by a white picket fence. Like Andre, Brandon is fifteen and presented to his local hospital with abdominal pain. He had been at a sports camp and had been unable to play, doubled over in agony. When Brandon's initial CT had shown that his appendix was normal, he was transferred to our service. Then he had gotten severe diarrhea. While we are waiting for the results of the stool studies to tell us just which of the many possible organisms is causing the trouble, he is being given IV morphine for pain and a stronger relative of Motrin called Toradol.

"We'll get him through this," Rishi reassures Brandon and his family. "The stool studies will take some time to come back, but while we're waiting he should ask his nurse for the morphine so at least we can keep him from being in too much pain. There's no need for him to try to tough it out or be heroic. All right, Brandon?"

In response, Brandon smiles seriously and nods. He is stiff in his bed and lies as still as possible as hands are shaken. Then Rishi and I step into the hall. Not long afterward, the nurse finds us in the conference room to inform us that Andre is again complaining of pain. It is an eight out of ten, ten being the worst pain imaginable. Brandon had rated his pain a six. I look up from the notes I am writing and glance toward Rishi.

"Has he tried Tylenol?" he asks the nurse.

"Not yet."

"Shouldn't we give him something stronger?" I ask.

Rishi gives a quick shake of his head, then says, "Why don't you check on him again?"

I grudgingly stand. From my own admittedly limited knowledge of their two cases, I can see no significant difference between Brandon's and Andre's complaints. At the moment, Rishi shakes his head so dismissively I bristle at the thought that it must be Andre's race, his relative poverty, that has relegated him to Tylenol instead of Toradol and opiates.

I knock and then open Andre's door partway, so I stand framed in the light from the hall.

"How's it going?" I ask.

Andre diverts his attention from the television to take a brief look at me.

"It's bad again," he complains. "It's like a nine out of ten."

I come forward the whole way into the room and stand by his side.

"Can I examine your belly?"

He nods, the handle of a plastic spoon protruding from between his lips. I slowly pull the bedcovers down to expose the area that I am meant to examine and then lift his oversized T-shirt and slide it up toward his ribs. His navel rises and falls slightly with each breath that he takes and I press my hands gently against his abdomen. He is still eating his ice cream, adapting to eat with his left hand as I am partially blocking his right.

"Does this hurt?" I ask him as I press harder, my right hand sinking in and then lifting up toward his spleen.

"It's awful," Andre winces, putting the spoon back in his mouth to lick the chocolate ice cream that remains. I am in a strange sense disappointed.

"All right," I say. "I'll leave you alone."

"Can't I have some medicine?"

"The nurse will get you some Tylenol. That should help with the pain. I still think on the whole that you're getting better."

"Why am I still pooping red?"

I stop, one hand resting lightly on the door frame, and turn to look back at Andre, who despite his query is still not looking at me. He is watching *Comedy Central* instead.

"I thought the nurses were checking all of your stools and there wasn't any blood."

"I don't know about that," Andre shrugs, his eyes still locked on the cartoon on the television screen where Barbra Streisand is involved in an altercation with the South Park boys. "But my poops are really red."

I report this back to Rishi, who once again assumes a professorial expression and steeples two fingers on which he rests his chin.

"Interesting. And the pain?"

"He says it hurts," I answer. "Now he's rating it a nine out of ten."

"What do you think?"

I know what he is asking me, so I tell him: "He didn't stop eating ice cream when I did my exam."

Rishi smiles and stands: "It can't hurt that bad then, can it?"

"You're right," I admit, and we are back on the same side again.

Rishi breezes into Andre's room. In one quick motion of a few overly large steps, he moves to stand directly between Andre and his television screen.

"I hear that you're still pooping red."

"Yeah." Andre seems almost surprised that Rishi should know this, despite having related as much to me only minutes before.

"Are they bright red?"

"They sure are."

"Are you eating lots of Jell-O?"

"What?" This time Andre appears not merely surprised but entirely dumbfounded.

"Jell-O," Rishi says again, raising his voice louder to carry over the sound of a Denny's commercial. "Do you like Jell-O?"

"I guess."

"Have you eaten any today?"

Andre considers this and seems to be searching painfully through his own internal records of what his day must have entailed. Finally, he says, "Yes."

"Was it strawberry?"

Andre's "yes" this time is revelatory as if by this divination Rishi is acting as shaman or oracle or sage.

"How many Jell-O's?"

Andre seems unsure, but he does a quick finger calculation and then ventures, "Six?"

Rishi reached his hands out before him with both palms up to the ceiling as if in offering.

"The Jell-O is turning your poop red, dude. No more Jell-O for you, all right?"

Andre nods almost as if compelled, entranced by what he certainly must think a somewhat strange prescription for a physician.

"All right."

"Fine then," Rishi finishes, and we both move around the foot of the bed and make for the door.

When we have closed it behind us, we hear Andre calling from the other side.

"Hey man!"

Rishi cracks the door and leans his head in.

"Do you have any Jell-O?"

Rishi sighs with the same self-deprecating attitude with which he might turn away street peddlers and prostitutes, a rejection and admission of defeat that at the same time suggests forgiveness and solidarity of a kind.

"No, dude. I don't have any Jell-O."

I was raised to believe that there are things that are worth fighting for. My father had chained himself to fences with others in protest during Vietnam and had lain down in front of the bulldozers years later at Love Canal. This last event I was old enough to remember, but too young to have been allowed anywhere near. I had been filled with a sense of urgency, an instinct to rush forward into the fray, but had found myself without any obvious affront against which to act. For a time I had considered not shaving my legs and becoming what we called crunchy and almost took a job the year after college to study capuchins and squirrel monkeys in Guyana, where I would have had to bathe in the river and pick my food from the trees. Instead I had chosen medicine to help people, as all medical school applicants proclaim almost in singsong, because it seemed a worthwhile cause with more reliable bathroom facilities.

Still, although we are a country that ranks unforgivably high in its health care disparities, if there was a battle raging to rectify this I was not anywhere in the vicinity of its front lines. The momentary indignation I had felt on Andre's behalf had been energizing but ultimately misdirected, and I had had to let it go. When we residents were confronted with glaring injustices, it was certainly our duty to report them, but this primarily took the form of contacting the Department of Social Services regarding the possible neglect or abuse of a child. Beyond summarizing our impressions of the family and particulars of the patient's medical management, no more was required. Even after a child had been removed from his or her family's custody, even if this child were to remain in the hospital for an extended period of time, the nuanced legal proceedings or outside investigations that might be ongoing were not information to which we ever were privy. Children simply disappeared for us when they left the hospital.

There would be, for example, later on in the year, four sisters between the ages of eight and twelve who lived for quite some months within our halls awaiting ultimate placement after removal from their own parents' care. This removal was prompted by their severe dietary deficiencies, malnourishment that was borne not directly of poverty but of adherence to a bizarre diet of their father's devise.

While the girls are on my service, all given the pseudonym Smith on their charts as well as on their doors for purposes of privacy, I care for them in strictly medical terms. I am concerned with the critically low levels of calcium circulating in their blood, an electrolyte that is only slowly being repleted, since it is at the same time being vociferously sucked up by their stunted and crooked bones. Although I would, from time to time, tuck the girls in at night, I have no clear notion of the abuses that took place. Despite my being included in an afternoon when the two eldest lined up their nail polish at the nurses' station and rounded up customers for their salon, I have no knowledge of what is ultimately said in family court. And though I want nothing more than to see them happy and free to play outside instead of trapped on a hospital floor, when I wave goodbye on the day they finally leave, I have no idea where they are ultimately going and with whom.

Toward the end of August, my mother stops for the evening on her way to a wedding up the coast. We do nothing in particular. We eat take-out burritos, sit on the couch in my apartment, and look over wedding proofs. It is all I have the energy for. She places the call to my grandmother and then hands over the phone. It is one of our family practices, guilt by physical approximation. I should call my grandmother other times, willingly and with spontaneity, while waiting for the bus to take me to afternoon clinic or while walking home at night. I should do this, but I don't. I call only when I am forced to, and even then, I do not dial the number myself.

The phone rings, and when she answers, her voice trembles with age but also with such excitement that I would like to take a knife to my own chest and cut out my beating heart. I am not a miracle, I would like to tell her. I am not a saint. I am not any kind of savior, although you might not know this had you ever listened to her recitation of my mediocre accomplishments, repeated with the same cadence and reverence with which a priest sings out the evening prayers. And it is for this reason that I never call, not because her hearing aid whistles or because it is tiresome to maintain her shaky concentration, but because by the very tone of her voice I see myself as she would have me and I know that I will never be as good as she believes me to be.

She is confused as we are talking or else she cannot hear my answers, so she asks me the same mundane questions several times. Finally, she says, "How are you liking your new job?" Although it will not make up for the distance I have been keeping, I know I have to lie.

What I tell my grandmother on the phone is that the hours are long. This is both a factual statement and an excuse, a three-year justification for all the phone calls I will fail to make. Beyond this I do not elaborate. I tell her my job is fine and that I am hanging in.

There are many things I have failed to tell the truth about over the years—my living arrangements with Daryl when we were still only dating, my opinions over the candidate she chose in the last presidential race—and so it is no stretch to also fail to mention that I hate my job. The way my feet feel when they have been trapped inside shoes and socks for more than a day's time is the way I feel about my life in more general terms. I am in need of a good airing out, but this is a difficult thing to actually say, and I fear I would not be understood.

There is one day in that first year I will look back upon as best representing how I actually felt for much of the time. On that day I am doing much the same job as I had been doing while at Children's with Rishi, but instead at the City Hospital a few miles away. I have had dental insurance for the first time in three years now that my residency has started, but in the past nine months I have not had the time to actually go to a dentist. When I do finally make an appointment, they find several cavities that I will need to come back to have filled. There is no room in my schedule that permits ducking out in the same way that others might leave a desk unattended. This is why I am postcall and having holes drilled into four of my teeth. After so many hours awake, it is a relief simply to let my eyelids fall shut. The whir of the drill as it penetrates my enamel and moves deeper to clean out the bacteria-filled hole is almost lulling if that is possible, blurred as it is with the continued buzz I am hearing that seems to come from inside.

The dental resident moves one finger along my gums and examines the work she has done. She then reaches for another gleaming tool from her tray and begins again. I do not open my eyes. As she leans over me, the lips behind her disposable paper mask must be moving. She likely thinks that paying attention, absorbing this careless narrative, is costing me nothing. She has no reason to know that there are depths of fatigue to which you can sink where even the act of processing sound is too much to ask. She is complaining about being on call from home to answer questions by phone on a Monday holiday that I did not even know existed. Despite this, I thank her profusely when I leave because she has done all of my fillings in one visit instead of two. She laughs and dismisses the compliment, but I know it would likely have taken another three months for me to find my way back again.

The bus that I take home passes right by Children's. As we cross the E line at Huntington, I see the Beetle convertible drive by. The top is back and the warm afternoon sun makes the curved yellow hood look even brighter, more cheerful than most inanimate objects can be. Seated side by side in the front are two of our chief residents, Mary Beth and Amanda. They are laughing, wearing sunglasses. Their dark hair is blowing backward, but gently, the way it only happens in television dramas or feature films. They look composed, confident, carefree in a way that I cannot remember ever being. Looking out the window, I suspect that my mouth is hanging open. I believe that it is, but I cannot tell for sure; I still cannot feel my face. What I want from my life in that moment is relatively simple. I want to be able to sleep in my bed on average once every twenty-four hours. I want to not slide from side to side in my thin scrubs on the orange plastic seat of a bus. I want, more than anything, to not be drooling in public.

This was a story that was laughed over later in the retelling, both by residents who knew Amanda and Mary Beth and also by those they had never met. In reality, though, it was not a funny story. It was sad and we laughed because we had to, because the subtext was too painful to ever speak out loud.

It is on a night not long after Andre has been sent home that I am left alone for the first time with Jane, a student in her third year of medical school. She has spent much of the last two years in a library and is just at the start of the clinical rotations that will take her through each field of medicine so that she can decide which of these she will choose to train in after she graduates. Each medical student is assigned to an intern and as such we have shared several calls. She has interviewed patients and done their exams. She has written up notes and helped with the endless electronic cataloging of data. In theory, Jane is meant to be learning from Rishi, since it is the third-years who have had more experience and more time to assimilate the things they have learned into salient talking points. In practice, much of the work that medical students are most helpful with falls under the direct purview of the intern with whom they are paired. Jane has put in an exemplary performance and is unprepossessing and sweet, yet I have until this point managed to use Rishi as a sort of shield. He filled in the empty spaces with his easy confidence and mock insults. In his presence I had been able to push away some of the suspicion, to file down a bit of the edge.

In another lifetime, one that feels just as distant as Mary Beth and Amanda's midafternoon jaunt from where I stand now, I had been Jane. I had been perky and industrious in my efforts to impress. In those minutes and hours before I was expected to be answering pages and rewriting orders and placating parents in the wake of a cockroach sighting, I had pored over textbooks and looked up relevant articles through the library website. I had made polished presentations at morning rounds. I had been smarter, in many ways, than I was now. Because of this, because Jane appears to me to be shiny and brimming with knowledge, I am scared that when we are alone she will turn to me with her innocent brown eyes and her oddly but perfectly smooth hair and ask me a question that I don't understand. It will not be one of those questions that can easily be fumbled through, looked up quickly, and passed off as a factoid that I had been in complete possession of only moments before but that had somehow been misplaced, like a pencil or a tube of Chapstick. I live in fear that she will casually inquire about a disease, the existence of which I am entirely unaware, most common in descendants of those immigrants who moved here from a country of which I've never heard and cannot find on a map, that causes its sufferers to exhibit symptoms described by words that I cannot even hope to spell.

Still, Rishi is in the ER seeing a new patient and Jane and I are by ourselves. In the conference room I am rechecking the dosing and necessary adjustments for Lovenox so that a five-year-old boy does not develop blood so thin that he will spontaneously begin to bleed.

"Is there anything I can do?" Jane asks.

I look at the clock and see that there are two more hours until our admitting responsibilities come to an end at midnight. Ideally, Sugar Call, the time when the day's blood glucose values for the diabetic patients are reviewed, happens every night around this time. Often, though, in the midst of admissions and other more pressing complaints, the session is pushed back until midnight closes in and the frustrated endocrine fellow calls in from home so that she can finally get to bed. But it is quiet, for once, and the admission waiting in the ER will come up to the floor before long; after that happens, it will be hard to find another lull during which to break away.

"Can you round up the bedtime sugars and write them on the board?"

"Sure," Jane says and practically flies off her seat to gather the numbers.

At this point in the year, before more of the system becomes computerized, this still means tramping up and down hallways and sometimes even to different floors to flip through the bedside charts that are hanging outside each patient's door. There are at almost all times a handful of new diabetics on the service, thin children who were well until they began experiencing excessive thirst, tiring quickly, and getting up several times in the middle of the night to go pee. These newly diagnosed type I diabetics stay in the hospital for two or three days while their parents learn how to check blood sugars and draw up insulin into thin syringes. They stay in the hospital while their blood sugars are slowly adjusted to a more acceptable range. Then they are sent home with their glucometer and their testing strips, their insulin needles, and a phone number to call every night. They are sent home and their parents continue the work where we left off.

Jane returns after a short time and writes the name of the first patient on the board. She makes columns for each of the times at which blood sugars are usually done: before breakfast, lunch, and dinner, before bedtime, and between two and four a.m. To the left of the numbers and just under the child's name, Jane writes the insulin regimen the child is on. The shots are typically given before breakfast, dinner, and bedtime. While in the hospital, patients may also get a shot to correct a high blood sugar before they eat lunch, but the goal is to find a combination of long- and short-acting insulin that will make this unnecessary, that will allow the child to have adequate coverage without having to be given a shot while at school.

Jane finishes with her chart of the four patients who are currently on the service.

"Should we go through it before we page Marta?" I ask.

"Sure," Jane answers and steps to one side so that I can see the whole board. Her short white coat is buttoned and the pockets bulge out, overstuffed with laminated study cards, a reflex hammer, and a tuning fork.

"Let's just start at the top," I suggest. "Where do you think we need to do better?"

Jane circles the value representing this child's blood sugar at lunchtime, which had been in the high 300s when it should ideally have been less than 150.

"He needs more coverage in the middle of the day."

"Good," I tell her. "How do we do that?"

There is a pause and then I say, "Which of the two types of insulin he's getting is more long-acting?"

"The NPH."

"Right," I say. "So we'll go up a little on his morning dose. He's getting 2½ right now. Should we just go to 3?"

"Okay."

Jane and I continue working for fifteen minutes more. When we have finished, the board is littered with our changes, brown numbers circled in red and the changes in the insulin doses written down in blue.

I page the endocrine fellow to the conference room phone.

"Why don't you take the call when it comes in?" I say to Jane. "Everything you need is up on the board."

Just then the phone rings and I press the button to activate the speaker.

"Hello?" Jane says. From the dusty black plastic cover of the telephone, a voice answers, "Hi."

Jane outlines for Marta the changes she would like to make to each patient's daily insulin dosing and at each step the fellow says that she agrees. She tells Jane that she has done a good job. Although Marta cannot see Jane's smile, it is obvious from her voice that it is there. I pass the new insulin order forms I have been filling out to let Jane sign them first and then I add my own name just below hers. Just as quickly as that brief moment of assurance and competence had come to me, it is gone, passed on to someone who would come next. I hold on to it for just another moment, that feeling of ownership, and then I let it go.

Feeders and Growers

I wake up and it is Thursday and it is December and somewhere on the other side of the door a baby is being born. When my eyes open, I do not know for how long I have slept. The two pagers I carry with me are lined up just below my pillow, but even so I fumble, pressing buttons with clumsy fingers while the shrill notes continue their wailing demand to be heard and answered. I think this must be what it is like to be crazy, to listen to voices that won't ever be quelled, to be filled to the brim with such a noise that it seems to come from inside, rattling your skull until you believe that your ears must start to bleed. Finally, my thumb connects with the proper button and I am rewarded with a quiet that is not silence, for there is no such thing within any hospital even at three in the morning. Still, it is some measure of blessed relief.

With the small bullet of plastic and electronics grasped in one hand, I allow myself just one more moment, the space of three measured breaths, and then I know that I have to turn over. I will myself into action. The thin but heavily starched sheet that had been covering me slides stiffly to one side as I roll onto my hip and drive an elbow into the center of the pillow to prop myself higher. I know it is only seconds that all this has taken, and I breathe as I slide my feet into my shoes and pull the door aside to burst into the hall.

This was my second rotation through a neonatal intensive care unit during the six months I had been a pediatric intern, but unlike the NICU next door to Children's—a vast service onto which many of the high-risk deliveries in the state were funneled when educated couples of a higher social class sought out the very best—this place was different. The patients who are wheeled through these doors are the uninsured, the newly immigrated, the teenagers. These women do not live in Wellesley or Brookline or Newton, but instead share an apartment with cousins in Mattapan or Dorchester or along Centre Street. When these women go into labor, they count out change for the bus while the time between the contractions becomes shorter and shorter.

When they arrive in triage, their clothes are stripped, their abdomens are exposed, and their stretch marks are covered by wide bands of cloth to hold the monitors in place. While the speakers spit out the gallop of a fetal heartbeat, IVs are inserted, quickly and with the minimum of fuss, and needles are pressed deep into their backs. These women do not know what questions to ask or perhaps they do not have the words in English with which to ask them. They sign their names on consent forms that have been printed in their own languages but which they still may not have the skills to read. They still somehow nod when it is expected of them, whether or not they understand what is being said. They moan deeply and in hushed, embarrassed tones as they hunch forward and pull their legs back into the air.

Entering a delivery room, I glance at the mother's bed only long enough to gauge how much time I have and then I turn my back. I wave my fingers through the air over the instruments I may be called on to use. I make note of where the bulb suction has been placed and reach my right hand out as if to grab it, practicing the movement so that it can be made quickly and in one fluid motion as soon as there is a need. I snap the laryngoscope blade open to make sure the tiny light illuminates and twist the bulb to ensure it will not come loose and fall into the infant's airway, that it is tightly held in place.

Ideally, my page should have told me more than the bare minimum of whether the delivery was vaginal or cesarean, information I glean from the room number and the two letters, LD for labor and delivery instead of OR, that were set before it. The page might have said VAC for vacuum or, less obliquely, FORCEPS. But there is nothing you can learn from a few abbreviated words flashed across the pager's small display that will ever prepare you to walk into the room. The smell of it hits you first, the metallic taste of blood that stings the back of the throat, the sweat, and all the things that you have never smelled before and consequently cannot call by their names; all of this is overlying disinfectant, rubber and plastic, and the salt of tears. Only after you have swallowed the taste of iron can you take in the jumble of bodies, the obstetricians crouching at the base of the bed, and the nurses standing ready beside them, their voices fighting to be heard over the infomercial or the talk show host blaring from the television suspended in one corner of the ceiling, which no one has had the forethought to switch off.

Sometimes the pager spits out small block letters that spell out MEC, which means that the amniotic fluid has been stained with meconium, the product of the first bowel movement, which should not be allowed to enter the infant's lungs when he or she emerges. Once the thin fluid is sucked into the airspaces, the potential damage is done; the resulting inflammation may cause breathing difficulty. There is no way to predict in those moments before the breath is taken how much of this fluid will be inhaled. So there is no way to predict which infants will later gasp for air and need oxygen or some other kind of support. It is not safe to leave any of them alone. Until that child screams, signaling that the opportunity to intervene has ended, the plan is always to insert a tube just below the vocal cords to suck the meconium out.

The first time I have to perform this act is in the middle of the night. The senior resident I am with looks like he should be wearing Birkenstocks and have a surfboard strapped to the roof of his hybrid car. Bret appears relaxed, and although I cannot entirely follow suit, I do not throw up while we are waiting, so I count this as a victory. He attaches the meconium aspirator to the suction tubing and I turn an oxygen valve. When the stunned and silent newborn is placed before me on the warmer, I am too gentle with the head and it slips to the side beneath my gloved fingers before I grasp the skull firmly and thrust two fingers into her tiny mouth to reveal a small ridge of gums and behind these the obstruction of her tongue. Then I press the blade of the laryngoscope against the pink taste buds, slipping the tube in place and nodding once. While I hold the endotracheal tube steady against the hard roof of the infant's mouth, Bret connects the aspirator and covers the open hole on the side of this cylinder, closing the loop and extending the suction down below. I pull back on the tube as the brown fluid is withdrawn. With my hand upon the small chest, I feel the newborn take in her first breath.

Afterward I called my mother while walking from the hospital to the T. I tried to explain what it felt like, standing there in waiting with the laryngoscope in my hand while the pregnant woman struggled to watch me save her child, the urgency in the obstetricians' voices cutting through the language barrier. If this woman had looked in my direction, she might have mistaken me for a child, except that she was little more than a child herself.

"Did you give the Apgars?" my mother asked when I had finished, referring to the score an infant is given to indicate how well (or poorly) it is doing. These are the numbers, along with weight and length, that parents tend to remember and brag about later on.

"I intubated in the delivery room," I told her in response, because that was the big thing, that was my victory, and I wanted her to share it.

My mother is a clever woman, she is a counselor and sincere, which together is a rare and wonderful combination. But then she asked me again, "Did you give the Apgars?"

So I told her, "Yes," and we hung up as I pulled open the door at the Hynes station and then walked underground.

She had missed the buildup, the heightening of tension, the years and years of storyline that was medical school and morning rounds and pagers that go off every twenty minutes between one and four a.m. There was no way for her to understand that what made it real to me that I was a doctor was not that I administered a routine assessment of the infant's coloring or muscle tone. I felt like a doctor because it was *my* back that blocked the new mother's view of the child she had waited for. It was *my* arm that she peered under to catch a glimpse of hair or hand while I used strange instruments to keep the child alive. *I* was the final hurdle before the baby could be placed within her arms, and it was in these motions that I found my authority: in the right-handed scoop and then suspension of an infant in the air while tossing wet and bloodied blankets aside with my left, and in the walking away from the reunited mother and child when the work was done and both were safe again. This was where the most frightening power and responsibility lay, this departure, and because it is one of the hardest things to teach, it is not an easy thing to learn. It is far easier to memorize the mandated emergencies, the conditions where it is imperative to move. It is why in that first year we quelled the urge to run, to rescue, to intervene, whenever our pagers rang. We had not yet learned when it is safe to triage, which requests could wait until the sandwich was eaten or the much-needed visit to the bathroom was completed. We could not yet tell whether to stay or go.

* * *

In the NICU, even after the shifts begin to blend together and some degree of comfort is finally reached, a page that signals a delivery means that it is time to run. The tiled corridor stretches before me and I rush past the open doors to my right without stopping until I reach the number I am headed for. The door is closed. Although I knock before pushing at the handle, I do not wait for acknowledgment before going in. Tiffany has gotten there before me, the creases from her pillowcase visible on one flushed cheek, and she is standing in the corner behind the warmer, pulling open the plastic packaging of the suction bulb and letting it fall (without touching it) onto one corner of the miniature raised bed.

"What's up?" I ask, waving a hand beneath the warmer's lights to ensure that the heat is on.

She shrugs: "I just walked in."

I pull a pair of purple gloves from the box tacked onto the wall and busy myself, helping Tiffany prepare things while we wait for the charge nurse to find a moment to tell us what we have been called in for.

We finish quickly, and when the nurse still does not look up from her clipboard, I hover behind her for a moment and then ask in a low voice, "What do we have?"

"Are you pediatrics?" she asks but does not yet turn.

"Yes."

"Give me just a sec."

She counts the instruments on the sterile table in front of her, bouncing her finger through the air, and then marks something down before she takes a step toward me.

"She's at thirty-four weeks, presented in premature labor five days ago. She has mag on board."

This is how things are condensed, sentences short enough to breathe in the space between the contractions, in the ringing vacuum of sound that punctuates the shrillness of the laboring woman's voice. I accept this information and move back to the warmer with Tiffany and the nurse who has come to join us from the NICU. There is something missing from the synopsis, as there always is, but as we mumble softly in our corner I cannot quite place what it might be.

I turn again to watch, trying to gauge from what is visible of the crowning head just how much longer it will be.

The woman, Rita, is crying. There is a man beside her, which I notice because it is significant and unfortunately rare, and I think how different this tableau that I am now a part of is from the first delivery I had been to that day, the sobbing fourteen-year-old and her mother, a room devoid of men. The girl had arrived too late for an epidural and she screamed as the tears were squeezed from her eyes.

"I can't do this."

"Yes you can," the OB told her from below.

Her mother remained seated in the chair beside the bed, a crossword puzzle in one hand and a pencil in the other.

"I don't want to," the laboring child cried.

The OB spoke more sharply this time: "It doesn't matter what you want right now, Janet. You have to push. You have to push now."

The girl shook her head and closed her eyes. Finally, her mother lowered the puzzle and stood.

"Janet," she said, her face still absent of expression. "It's time for this baby to come out. Now do what you've been told."

Then she walked out of the room, taking her puzzle and her pencil with her. Later I would learn that the girl had wanted an abortion but had been told she would have to go to court because her mother refused to give consent. At that point the matter had been dropped and the fetus had grown to term.

In the room I am now standing in, there is screaming. There are tears. But the voice that is raised is not that of a frightened child brought into adulthood far too soon. This voice is familiar, although not because I have met this woman before; I recognize it as the roar that comes from a mother who has made this choice deliberately, who wants this child and is willing to fight for it. Then there is no time to think on it further because the infant's head is out, then his shoulder, and he is lifted limp and is not breathing as he is carried toward us.

I stand aside to let the OB resident place the newborn onto the swath of blankets we have opened on the warmer.

"Mom has hep C," she whispers. With those few words, I take in the meaning of the scene, the drugs this woman must have taken, the needles that would have pierced her veins.

"How much methadone is she on?" I ask to determine how sleepy I should expect the child to be, how much of this medically prescribed oral replacement for heroin he has been exposed to during the weeks of gestation after his mother came in to get clean.

"Sixty," the OB resident says and then slips away, leaving the head of the warmer open for me to move into place.

The first time I had encountered this, I was not thirty yards from where I was now standing. I was gowned and gloved, wearing a gauze-like blue cap on my head. On the table of the operating room was the pregnant patient at approximately twenty-four weeks gestation, although her dates could have been off in either direction. She was high as they tried to insert the needle into the small of her back for the spinal anesthesia needed to perform her cesarean section. Despite the blood pooling between her thighs or else because of it, she was too agitated for the needle to be safely inserted between her vertebrae.

The pregnant woman was upset; she had too many drugs and too much alcohol on board to be able to take in the calming voice of the OR nurse, the instructions to sit still. It was not alcohol that brought the labor on, although this exposure was certainly not a kindness to her growing child. Instead, it was the lines of coke she snorted in bathroom stalls and strangers' bedrooms, off of dirty kitchen countertops and the back of her own hand, that had caused the placental vessels to clamp down. Even if she had not gone on that particular binge, the baby would have come out too small; even without that last snort of blow, the infant would have suffered both before and after it was born. But the pregnant woman had taken one last snort and then she had started to bleed.

"How could I do this?" she yelled as she thrashed back and forth and needed to be held down. "I did this to my baby. What kind of a mother does this to her baby?"

No one said anything; no one gave her an answer because it was not the sort of truth that could change the thing that was about to begin. The placenta had pulled away from the wall of her uterus and all of the blood that should have been feeding the fetus was leaking out. This woman was dying, and delivering her baby was the only way she could be saved. She was put to sleep because she could not sit still. While she lay unconscious, the baby was cut out.

I was the only one from the NICU in the operating room when the baby emerged, the usual resuscitation table standing empty, with the personnel gathered just across the hall in a better-equipped treatment room. I was responsible for waiting while the obstetrician cut and clamped the umbilical vessels. I held my arms out before me, draped in warmed sterile blankets that had also been laid across my chest. I knew that the blankets were placed in this way to act as a cocoon of sorts, that the child would be placed in my arms, and that I would then fold them up to my body, enveloping her small form and scuttling quickly out the door and through another to deposit her beneath the radiant warmer before her core temperature had a chance to fall. I knew that she would be tiny, but I did not know how tiny, that my outstretched arms were too far apart for her premature but also stunted form, and that when she was gently dropped upon me, I would not be able to register the weight. I knew that she would need to be intubated, but I did not realize that it would take more than half a dozen attempts by my senior resident and the attending, sliding the tube down and then bagging, waiting for the oxygen saturation on the monitor to respond to the small gusts of oxygen we were delivering or for the carbon dioxide monitor to change color as the baby breathed out, only to see no change at all, to have the tube removed and then replaced so many times that it occurred to me that perhaps it was not the tube placement that was the problem but rather the fact that her immature lungs could not extract the precious gas that her body's tissues so desperately needed.

The infant's oxygen saturation remained stubbornly in the mid-60s instead of climbing to 100, but she did not die there in that room. She was taken into the NICU. She was given round after round of epinephrine. In the recovery room her mother was extubated and woke up, but was still so combative that she needed to be sedated again. There was no next of kin listed on her paperwork. There was no one who could give us permission to stop. The baby was gray the way that meat is when it has already gone off, when the rotting has truly set in, but her heart kept on beating, so we could not declare her dead.

The attending and the other resident coded the twenty-four weeker for more than six hours before they finally called it. There was no ringing of chimes or moment of silence. Things simply went on. The small gray form that had been the center of such furious energy was covered over and people walked away. Because her mother was still unconscious and they did not know what else to do, and because the hospital admission paperwork has a space to indicate a religion and her mother's papers said that she was a Catholic, they had called in the chaplain. They had kept the ventilator and the fluids and the pressors all going while she was baptized, namelessly, so that she might not be punished for her mother's sins.

Tiffany and I are both aware that the methadone is not the reason the newborn girl before us is not crying, or why her arms are flung flat on either side of her instead of bent tightly to her sides. It is because of the magnesium that her mother had been given to slow down her contractions, to give her more time inside, precious days and hours during these last weeks to get as much growing done as possible.

Her chest is rising, but only slightly. I discard the bulb with which I've cleaned her mouth and nose and reach for the oxygen mask as Tiffany and the NICU nurse continue to rub her from head to toe, trying to trigger that first deep intake of air, the one that opens up the lungs and makes each breath after it easier to draw in. I hold the mask over her face, making a seal around her mouth and nose, and the green bag inflates to signal that oxygen is flowing. Tiffany places a finger on her palm, but she does not grasp it. She lifts one of her small arms above her and then lets it fall. Her small body is turning from simply pale to blue. Our eyes meet and I take the bag in my right hand, still holding the mask in place. I squeeze it and feel the air leaking out beneath the soft lips of the mask, blowing across the infant's cheeks instead of entering her lungs. I reposition the mask, placing three fingers along her jawline, and with my index finger and thumb I make a C to hold all sides of the mask tight up against her face. I squeeze again. Her chest rises nicely; I squeeze a few more times.

Behind us, her mother is still crying, "Why can't I have my baby? I want to hold my baby now."

She cannot focus, cannot begin to take in the activity surrounding her newborn daughter, can only think that she has been taken from her and in her guilt cannot dismiss the fear that she will not be given back.

The father has let go of Rita's hand and is standing close beside us, taller than any of us three, towering in the narrow space between Tiffany and myself. He is in a T-shirt and jeans. His nails, I notice as he reaches a finger out to point at his daughter, are caked with dirt.

In the first daze of fatherhood he has also failed to notice the urgency with which we are working, the puffs of air that are being forced into his child.

"She's beautiful, Rita." He looks over his shoulder to tell the woman who is not his wife, who is in fact still married to someone else. "She's perfect. We did something good."

I am amazed by this, as I always am, this blind assumption that the birth of any child is somehow miraculous even when disaster lurks so near. In the NICU right now, there is a child born early at twenty-seven weeks, feet first into a toilet, the placenta like a counterweight on the dirty tile beside the bowl. His mother had passed out not from blood loss but from cocaine. It was another woman in that apartment, also high, who had just enough presence of mind to realize that when there is a baby in a toilet, you should dial 911. Unfortunately, though, she did not have enough of her wits about her to lift the baby out, so she was still in the toilet when the paramedics arrived. It was a miracle, they said, that she was not born head down. It was a miracle she didn't drown. And my stomach tightens as I turn away and curse this world where we accept such half measures as signs of some divinity, where we praise the heroin user for switching to methadone or the cocaine addict for cutting down on the blow. It is not that I do not recognize the enormity of these achievements in the face of an addiction, but I have come to know in the last six months of this residency that there are worse things than not being born.

In the delivery room the baby cries at last, the sound of it muffled by the dome of the mask upon her face. I pull away and we are still for a moment, hands ready. Tiffany flicks the sole of her foot. Her lips part to reveal the empty rows of her gums. She screams with frustration and despair as all newborn children must. It is a sound that all new parents need to hear, this admonition and this warning. The cry echoes against the cold tile of the walls and floor, demanding that henceforth she should be handled with more care and gentleness than the ordeal she has just endured. And the sharpness of this cry is a shard of green glass that is spun long with razor thinness, and it enters those for whom it is calling just behind the left ear, lodging in the hollow between the mandible and mastoid, a reminder, a pact, and one that has been made with the scent of blood heavy in the air.

She is breathing, but her tone is still poor, her arms and legs splayed and resting flat against the pink and blue striped towels beneath her. We will need to watch her closely, but there is nothing more that we can do for now, so there is time to explain things, if her parents are able to listen. Her mother keeps asking to hold her, over and over, and despite the fact that her queries have not been successful, she has not changed a single syllable, has not altered the inflection of her desperate plea. I think how this, too, is the drugs, this behavior, this most basic inability to try something new when what you are doing yields such an obvious absence of results.

It is necessary in talking with parents to start with something that is good. It is a moment that should not be skipped over, however more imperative all of the other sentences that will come after seem to be. Congratulations are given to the family of the child with Down syndrome because they have been blessed with a healthy boy. His presence should be cherished, completely and without question, for a few seconds at least. There will be many hours spent discussing the studies that will have to be done of his heart or how he may have difficulty holding his head steady or trouble feeding, but there should first be a time when the good is reveled in, when the joy is allowed to be complete.

"She's taking nice deep breaths," I tell this family, still with one hand resting lightly on the infant's head. "Her tone is still low; you can see that she's not really moving her arms or legs. That's because of the magnesium that you got, mom, to help stop your contractions. This will keep getting better. We just need to keep watching her for a bit before we wrap her up and let you hold her."

"Can I touch her?" the girl's father asks.

I cringe inwardly as I glance at his fingernails, but there is no way to refuse.

In the vacuum where my words should be, Tiffany comes to my rescue and says, "Of course."

I move my hand so that the NICU nurse can slip a knitted hat onto the girl's head and then she leaves. I step back to give the father room to take one of his daughter's small hands between his filthy index finger and thumb.

"She'll get antibiotics anyway," Tiffany whispers to me with a shrug, then asks, "Are you okay here?"

"Yeah," I say. "I'll bring her over when she's ready."

Tiffany turns toward the parents and explains what has to happen next: "She's doing very well, but she'll need to come to the special nursery, the NICU, because she was born so early. We want to make sure she has the best nurses taking care of her. I'll just go and make sure they're ready for her once you're done here."

"Will we be able to visit her?" his mother asks.

"Anytime and for as long as you like," Tiffany replies and moves away. She pulls aside the curtain that is hung in front of the door to make a sort of foyer. The curtain falls back and I hear the door open and then swing shut.

"I want to hold my baby," Rita says, and it has started again, this skipping record that she cannot help but play.

It is not that I am being cruel or even that there are checklists that must be run down. The infant must be weighed; she needs erythromycin ointment over her eyes and a shot of vitamin K in her thigh. More importantly, though, while she is lying on the warmer I can see her from anywhere in the room, can see the rise of her narrow chest, can watch for the outline of her ribs that would mean she's pulling too hard and might be tiring. Her parents do not realize that she still looks far from well and wouldn't be able to identify the signs if she was taking a turn.

"Of course you do," I tell her in reply, trying to make the tone of my voice both sympathetic and resolute, since I suspect she is not really listening to my words. "But she needs to start moving more on her own first, and until she does, I need to be able to see all of her, uncovered like she is. If we take her off the warmer, she'll get too cold."

I reach down to take her small hand in mine, a hand that should be a fist but isn't. The fingers close weakly around my own and I point this out to her parents, another small improvement, another piece of good.

While we wait, I have time to look through Rita's chart. Her history is documented there, all the urines that had tested positive for opiates, the last of these in October, only ten weeks before her baby was born. Methadone, I have learned, has a structure that is different enough from heroin that it is not picked up by a tox screen, so this last positive urine test was also the last time she was high, the last time she had a needle in her arm or between her toes. These are things it is important for me to know, but it is also difficult because there is information that is missing. Although the chart tells me that this mother denied using alcohol or benzos or cocaine while she was pregnant, it does not tell me how much the father knows. He may not know that she has hepatitis C; he may not even know about the methadone or the heroin or how many children she has had before. These are the sort of secrets that are kept even from partners; they are the reason that sex and even love and marriage do not bring full truth. And so there are things that need to be talked about that cannot be brought to the surface here. There will have to be stolen moments and hurried and lowered voices before I can find out just how much this man has been told.

As I write my own note in the infant's chart, deducting the points for respiratory effort and tone and color at one minute and at five and ten, the nurse is securing her name bands around one ankle and one wrist. Her father leans closer to read the printed text and looks at me with alarm.

"That's not her name. That's Rita's husband's name. I want her to be called after me."

"She'll have her mom's name on her records for as long as she's in the hospital. You'll have to ask how it works when you fill out the birth certificate. I don't know anything about that."

"Can't you change it now?" he asks.

They used to do this. They used to make accommodations, and it seems like such a small thing to do for something that feels so big. But there were errors, with all the bundled babies in their matching white cotton shirts and the mothers in their dowdy frocks. It was hard enough to address the infant using the proper pronoun the first time you spoke with a family you had never met. In the end, it was too difficult to keep the stories straight, to remember who belonged to whom.

"It's his first baby. He's excited," Rita says as if this needs an explanation, which it doesn't, but she has also told me that he knows that she has had other children.

"Sure," I tell them. "It is exciting, but the rules are there so that we don't make mistakes."

"You don't have to apologize, honey," she tells me. Then, "I'm sorry. I know that you're a doctor. It's just that you look so young. What's your name again?"

"It's fine," I say, because she is right. "You can call me Meghan."

"Thanks."

"Does she have a name yet?" I ask her as I pause to fill in that space on my index card.

"The baby?" she asks.

"Yes, the baby," I nod.

"We're going to call her Myranda."

I go back to writing; as I do, I watch the nurse lift her onto the scale and note the extent to which she controls her head, the tightness of her hands. She is improving.

"She can hold her when you've finished," I tell the nurse.

Later, with my mother on the phone and my husband sitting nearby, this is where I start the story. These are the bits it is possible to share, because there has to be something you tell the people closest to you when they ask how your day was and because every time you say, "It was good," you are telling them a lie.

I am still writing when the OB shows her the placenta and explains which side was against her insides and what parts make up the bag the infant floated within. There is still a small stream of blood leaking from her vagina and the OB leans in to take a closer look.

"We'll just need to place a few stitches here to close up this tear," Rita is told. "I'll numb you up first."

The OB resident begins and I am still waiting for the newborn to come to the NICU with me. Her father is holding her now, the grimy fingertips leaving dark marks on the clean towels the infant is wrapped within. He is smiling, rocking his daughter from side to side. He is not looking at his child's mother as she is sewn up down below. This is something that happens, and there are fathers who follow their children to the nursery while the mother is in the OR with her abdomen still open wide. I let them drink in the small fingers and toes, the still closed eyes, and when some time has passed, I say gently, "How's mom doing?" to send them on their way.

"These stitches will dissolve on their own, so they don't need to be taken out." The OB resident is still leaning forward, between the woman's legs, as she says this.

"How long?"

"Sorry?" She does not look up, but continues passing the curved needle through the broken flesh.

"How long until it's good down there?" Rita pauses, waiting to be understood. More red fluid leaks out and runs down one buttock to join the pool in which she sits.

"The bleeding will get a little less every day," the resident tells her, but this is not Rita's question, and she tries again.

"How long for sex?"

I wish I could record this moment, because it is so inappropriately out of place. There are certain ways of doing things, lines that should not be crossed.

The OB resident does look up this time and says, I think fairly sharply, "You shouldn't have sex for at least six weeks. You need to give yourself time to heal."

On the phone, I say, "What was she thinking?"

I also say, "Where did that come from?"

Above my mother's and my husband's laughter, I say, "I'm sure if that baby's daddy was looking at the bloody mess between those legs, he would have been thinking, 'I've got to get me some of that.' And she's just forced such a large object out of her vagina that she's been torn in two. Is that really the time to think, gee, when can I be slammin'?"

And I think, but I do not say out loud in the delivery room or even later on the phone, "That child will be crippled by the family she is in."

Myranda is finally in her mother's arms. As the OB resident drops her needles in the red plastic wall-mounted container for sharps, she says, "If you're going to breastfeed, now is a good time to see if she'll latch on."

I feel my eyebrows raise, but it is not my place to disagree. The hospital policy says that as long as a former drug user is on methadone when her baby is born, as long as she is not HIV positive, she should be allowed to breastfeed if she wants to. The methadone is present in the breast milk, but not in concentrations significant enough to impact the course of the infant's withdrawal. This was something people had disagreed about, had fought and argued for, and although in the end there were no good answers, it was decided that consistency was what was of the most importance. One mother should not be told many different things. She should be supported and encouraged to bond with her new infant, should be told that her breast milk is absolutely the healthiest nutrition that she can give.

If it were my choice—and I know that it is not—this is not a woman I would want to breastfeed. She has hep C, which probably means that she shared her needles. She was using as recently as ten weeks before she gave birth. Her HIV test was negative when all of her prenatal labs were drawn, but that was hardly reassuring given that more recently still she had needles in her arms.

Later that night, in my call room, I open my copy of the latest Bret Easton Ellis and in it beautiful people are snorting cocaine in swanky bathroom stalls. They are popping Xanax and Klonopin; they are the chic on heroin and crystal meth. And somehow while I am reading I believe that it is possible to have drugged-up sex in limousines and not be punished for your sins. But that is not the world that Rita lives in. She has tears in her eyes when she tells me how much she misses her other daughter and son; how she tried to divorce her husband but did not know how to find out where he had gone; how her kids are smart, are doing well in school, so she left them with her mother when Myranda's father had to come down here to work so that they could finish out the school year. They would be together as a family once the summer came.

When she tells me all this, I am aware that she is lying. I ask her if her children are in her custody, and she tells me yes, they are. But the Department of Social Services (DSS) had taken these children away and they were with their grandmother because the state, and not their mother, thought that it was best. She told one of the nurses that she had sons and that Myranda was her first girl. She told the social worker that while DSS had been involved with her other children, they had cleared her. Yet despite these lies, they somehow *will* decide to clear her, after a home inspection, and this infant will remain hers.

When Rita has finished talking about her absent children I explain how Myranda will need to remain in the hospital for the weeks or even months that she is in withdrawal. The opium she is being given will be tapered off once she has been captured, once the necessary dosage has been reached, but it is early, she is only a few days old, and the methadone is in her fat stores and is only slowly being cleared. What she is experiencing is called neonatal abstinence syndrome, or NAS. It is not a short stay she has in front of her, but once she is eating and is cleared of any signs of infection from her prematurity and the difficulty of her labor, she will be safe to go to the regular pediatric ward upstairs. The general pediatric team will care for her until she is ready to go home. For now, she is being given oxygen and she has a feeding tube that has been slipped into her nose and down into her stomach to give her the calories that she needs to counteract the shaking chills and the diarrhea that are part of her withdrawal.

I sit with Rita while she talks though the guilt because, truth or lie, it is something that she needs to do. She is still pumping breast milk, for us to run through Myranda's feeding tube when at the end of each feed she stops sucking and falls asleep. Rita has been discharged. If she is using again, we have no way to know. The breast milk could be contaminated, but DSS has made their ruling and there is no way to stop her from feeding her daughter. As we talk, we keep our voices low. It is against every unwritten rule to wake an NAS baby, to make her fuss and cry and thus score higher in the nursing assessment of her symptoms, in which case her medication dosing would need to be increased. Infants who are held tend to do better, so I encourage Rita to take her in her arms. Next to where we are seated, a young mother of a former twenty-six-week infant shows off a new tattoo with her daughter's name. She has had time to get a tattoo but not the car seat required for the baby's release, and I take a deep breath to suppress my anger, trying to focus on what Rita has to say. Sitting there feels like listening to confession, draped in robes and seated behind an ornamental grille, dispensing Hail Marys and other chanted substitutions for atonement.

"What happens now?" Rita asks before they go, before Myranda is transferred to the regular inpatient team to continue her opium wean.

I tell her, "Well, she's off the oxygen and her lungs are doing fine on their own even though she was born just a little bit early. We've already talked all about her withdrawal. Aside from that, she's just a baby. She's still very small, but I know she'll do great. All of this is just normal stuff. She's a feeder and grower now."

Finally, when we have finished talking, she tells me, "Thanks, honey, for being so sweet."

And as Rita leaves to begin her drive home, there is a whisper in my ear from behind me, "Be careful or you'll become their pediatrician."

I turn to see my attending shrug knowingly and then walk away.

On the phone I rant and my mother asks me, "Why are you so angry?"

"I'm tired," I say, because I have been up for thirty hours straight.

"Can't you tell her that you'd be happy to see her in clinic as long as she stayed off the drugs?"

"No, because it's when she's on the drugs that we need to see her most. She can't be scared away."

"So are you going to keep being her doctor?"

"She never actually asked," I reply.

I will not be her pediatrician, it turns out. Myranda and her family will soon move away. And I am never really able to explain my anger to my mother. I am angry because the last time I was on the platform waiting for a train at Hynes, a man came up to me and asked me for a dollar. He was already inside; he did not need the money to get where he had to go. I said no because I did not have any money, but also because he was the father of one of the babies I had admitted earlier that day. Despite my scrubs and fleece hospital jacket, he did not recognize me. I am angry because you need a license to drive a car and own a gun and sell alcohol but not to have or raise a child. I am angry that I live in a country that cares so much for the rights of unborn children but gives so few resources for the stewardship of those children after they are delivered. I am angry about many things and wish I had the energy to see my way forward to someday making changes, even little ones, but at the end of the day, it is hard enough to stay awake.

Women's Troubles

I had not anticipated sex would be present in so much of what I was expected to do as a pediatrician. I thought of babies as being fairly androgynous for the most part, chubby and bald, with their clothing carefully color coded by parents desperate to avoid that awkward confrontation when a stranger mistakes their newborn boy for a girl or the other way around. I quickly learned that it was best to sidestep any potential mishaps before entering a patient's room by scanning the paperwork for the capital M or F, which was much more reliable than trying to make a guess based on the infant's first name.

But while infants were indeed a large part of the patient population for whom I was responsible during residency, it turned out that I also saw children and young adults up to twenty-one. Unlike the medical students who begin their pediatrics rotations terrified that they will forget to support a newborn's head and that it will somehow come right off, I had been handed enough slick and squirming infants in delivery rooms to know that they are relatively difficult to break; I have learned that their heads, while certainly too heavy for their neck muscles to control with any degree of finesse, are nevertheless stuck on pretty tight. It was the teenagers I was unprepared for, terrified of even, with their propensity for sullenness and outright lies, their inability to state in any simple and straightforward terms what was bothering them and why they needed to see a doctor. This is perhaps an unfair assessment of all people between the ages of thirteen and twenty-one, but as far as I was concerned that was all the more reason to be nervous about them. There was no way, standing outside of the room, to prepare for what was inside. There are seventeen-year-olds who have never even considered having sex and there are fourteen-year-olds with whom I have had to talk about breastfeeding and circumcision and how to find day care so that they don't have to drop out of school before finishing eighth grade.

It was the teenage girls in particular who were famous for dropping in a "by the way" at the end of a visit. This happened in the adolescent clinics at both of our hospitals and also in the ER, too often and inexplicably at three a.m. The patient is a fifteen-year-old girl, or she is sixteen or seventeen, and her chief complaint, the thing she told the triage nurse when she first came in, is that she is having aches and pains. I talk to her and find out that she is having mild headaches and a runny nose. Her throat is scratchy. She is a bit more tired than usual and is eating a little less.

"Are you still able to go to school?" I ask to find out just how severe these symptoms are.

"Not really."

"What does that mean? Did you go to school today?"

"Yes," she might tell me reluctantly.

"Did you go to school yesterday?"

"Yes."

"When was the last time you took Tylenol or Motrin for the pain?"

"I haven't taken anything."

"You haven't taken anything for three days?"

If she shakes her head, I am usually convinced that she does not need to be here.

I tell her that long warm showers or a humidifier can sometimes make breathing a little easier and help to clear out her sinuses and that she can take a decongestant if the runny nose is really bothering her, but to be careful because many of those medicines can make you drowsy. I do not tell her anything that I don't consider common sense. At the start of my residency, these conversations were difficult. I felt it was a failure on my part somehow to not have thought up anything more profound to say. But then Daryl got sick for the first time since we were married. He skulked around the apartment with a drippy nose rubbed raw by Kleenex, mouth hanging open so that he could breathe, until I hand delivered two tablets of cold medicine and a glass of water and told him to drink them down. At that point I realized that not all teenagers (or even adult physicists) have developed their common sense and that these instructions need to be made clear. They need to learn that there are times when they will be sick and that growing up is learning to take care of yourself; there will not always be someone else to do it for you.

Sometimes the visit ends this way. But not infrequently when we have finished this last piece of the conversation, the teenager drops in the "by the way" casually, almost as if she hopes that I will not notice, that she will still be allowed to leave with the last words being those of reassurance, that nothing at all is really wrong.

"By the way," she might mention, "I've also been having a smelly discharge from my vagina for about a week."

Whether I am in clinic or the ER when this happens, I have other patients waiting. It is hard not to blame this girl, who, despite having breasts larger than mine and in all likelihood more sexual experience than I would ever want, is still a child. It is not only my time that she is wasting, for there are other children and their parents in the rooms to either side. It is a sort of trap that I fall into all the time, but it is not one that I can simply free myself from and run. I have to stay.

I start over with my history taking, knowing that this visit will take another forty minutes at least, because she will need more questioning and an internal gynecologic exam as well. We review her sexual history, her lifetime number of partners, the age she was when she first had sexual intercourse, the percent of time she uses condoms, which often turns out to be not at all. She is, in nearly all of her subtle incarnations, not currently on the pill.

Once I had asked, "Are you on the pill?" to an overweight twenty-one-year-old who had come into the clinic for a pregnancy test.

And she had responded, "What?" with an expression that indicated such complete lack of understanding that I was shocked enough to not know how to proceed.

"There is a pill that you can take every day that has the same hormones that your own body produces," I said as if to jog her memory. "It stops your ovaries from releasing an egg each month so you don't get pregnant even if you are having sex."

"I didn't know that."

There are young teenagers and there are old, and this distinction has nothing at all to do with age. I was a young teenager. When I was brought into the ER by my mother at age eleven for an injury to a toenail, the resident began asking me questions about sex that I did not even begin to comprehend. It was not that I was unaware of where babies come from; I was three when my brother was born, and he was still strapped into his infant seat in the back of the car when I asked my mother the question that she thought she had at least a decade more to prepare for. Even still, being able to shock my grandmother at the age of four with an accurate description of how the sperm come to find the egg did not mean that I would, when faced with the possibility of sex during my own teenage years, have any idea how I should feel. Maybe a talk from my own pediatrician would have left me more empowered and less afraid, but I cannot really blame her for not asking. It is a difficult conversation to have at the best of times, and even the smallest of distractions—the intrusive page or knock on the exam room door—can make it impossible to carry out with grace. In such a situation it is easy to say nothing. This young type of teenager can be hard to talk to, and while they—like I was—might be confused and tormented and moved to write moody and ultimately bad poetry, they are most likely safe.

Old teenagers, in contrast, actually do those things without knowing how to feel, and those actions cannot be ignored. Those awkward, sticky moments in the backseats of used cars or underneath the bleachers have very real implications for their health and safety, so the conversation becomes one that I cannot avoid. The parts of their lives that should be the most private—the heartbreak, the rejections, the transformation of each new beginning into something stale and sordid that will last too long but then will eventually and precipitously end—were my job to unearth and expose. And when I had done that, nodding sympathetically while listening to the litany of sex acts and number of lifetime partners, it was my responsibility to deliver judgment of the sort rained down by television evangelists and Fox News anchors. I was meant to soothe only then to wound.

It would have been disingenuous to say, "I know what you are feeling," because it simply was not true. In other situations it bothered me less, the distance between my own experience and what my patients were going through. It was not conceivable that I could ever really understand how the asthmatic feels when his lungs close up or how the diabetic copes with the encroaching darkness when her sugar bottoms out. Such experiences are emotionally charged, certainly, maybe even as much as sex, but they are also more easily attributed to physiology, to something that is broken and needs to be repaired. In those instances it felt like it was enough to be able to fix the problem. So it was straightforward by comparison to encourage the children with diabetes or asthma to make smart decisions, to take their insulin every day or use their inhalers regularly according to their asthma action plan. It was far more difficult to tell fragile teenagers, desperate for love and affirmation, that in seeking out these things they so deserve they are somehow doing something wrong. It was a task that I found nearly impossible, always afraid that I would be challenged, asked, "What do you know about it?" to which I would be forced to answer, "I don't know anything at all."

It is a rare occurrence, but I sometimes find myself inside a room with a girl who is not unlike myself. Carrie is a college student. She is white. She comes into the clinic at the start of summer wearing a knee-length cotton skirt and a tank top covered by a loose and colorful blouse. Her toenails are painted a soft pink and on one toe there is an intricate metal ring. Her flip-flops are decorated with shiny blue sequins and beads and there is a Greenpeace patch stitched onto her bag.

"I didn't shave my legs," she apologizes, later and unnecessarily, once her feet are up in the stirrups. Because I know that she cannot see me through the sheet that is draped across her knees, I let myself smile.

"I need to be tested for everything," she tells me, apologetic again.

She does not have any idea what she is asking, the long list of swabs and stains and blood tests this would entail. She is only doing as she was told.

"What sort of symptoms do you have?"

"My ex-boyfriend saw something on his private parts."

"On his penis?" I ask.

"Yes," she answers. She does not use the forbidden word.

"Is there just the one lesion?"

"I think so." Carrie does not seem convinced and I try to imagine the conversation between them, how indignant he must have sounded then, how his anger left no room for Carrie to defend herself.

"What does it look like?"

"I don't know," she answers helplessly.

"Is it painful?"

"I don't know."

She cannot tell me the color, the shape, if the area is ulcerated or raised, if it gives off an odor, if it has grown or shrunk.

"When was the last time the two of you had sex?"

"Almost two weeks ago. I went to visit him. Then we broke up. He called to tell me that I needed to get myself checked out and tested for everything to find out what he has."

"What did his doctor say?"

"He hasn't been to one. He said that whatever it is must have come from me, so I should be the one who has to go get seen."

"That's a little ridiculous," I tell her, because I can see the weight of all this pressing on her, the assumption that this is somehow her fault. It is ridiculous that she should be made to feel this way, for a bump that may in the end turn out to be a pimple or something similarly unimportant, and it is ridiculous that I will order thousands of dollars of testing because his penis is not there in front of me and I cannot see what the problem is most likely to be.

"I know." She gives a half smile and I can tell that she is embarrassed but also that she was too scared to leave it in his hands.

I should refrain from commentary, but I cannot help but say, "That's not an okay thing for him to do to you. Maybe it's a good thing you two broke up."

"Yes," she says. "I think so, too."

Carrie has not been with anyone else since she and her ex-boyfriend got together. Although they did not use condoms all the time, she tells me that they had both been tested for STDs before the first time they had unprotected sex. I tell her that I will look carefully everywhere to see if I can find anything that she may have missed. We will send off tests for gonorrhea, chlamydia, and syphilis, but those results take some time to come back. Also, although HIV does not cause external lesions, we can arrange for counseling so that she can be tested. I try to be reassuring because I know that in the absence of any visible lesion I will not be able to give Carrie an answer today.

I had fumbled a bit when I first started doing pelvics. Even though each time I explained what I was doing before I did it to make my patients less uncomfortable, I don't think I ever really put anyone at ease since I was not at ease myself. Now, as my intern year was drawing to a close, I had done enough of them to dispel the lingering sense of mild discomfort. As with all things, repetition eventually dulls the fear. With her feet up in the stirrups, I am relaxed as I have Carrie move her backside down on the exam bed until she feels that she will fall off. Her legs are angled in so that her knees rest up against each other. I do not want to have to pull her knees apart myself; however gentle I may be, it is still an invasion of a kind. Instead, I hold my hands out to indicate where I want her knees to be and ask her to let her legs fall open until they are resting against my palms. I wait until she is repositioned before I lift the thin white sheet to take a look.

I tell her that everything looks normal, both because it does and because it is something every young woman needs to hear. Even if I had found something, I hope I would have told her that everything was normal except for that one small spot. For some patients with genital lesions, I would have found a little value in shocking the senses, but it is clear that Carrie is not a girl who needs to be any more scared than she already is. Most important, though, I do not see anything that is cause for concern. I continue with the exam and gather the samples that I need to send off to the lab. When we are finished, I take her down the hall to the office where the HIV counseling is done and where, because of a new grant, testing is done by a cheek swab instead of blood.

"I'll call you on your cell when the results come back," I explain before we part. "But I'm sure that it will all be fine."

And it will be fine. Carrie's testing all comes back negative. Saying goodbye to her, I have a vision of the girl I once had been, but it is no longer me. I realize that it is because I had seen myself in her that I had so easily provided both reassurance and the necessary censure. The words that at other times stuck in my mouth—the condemnation of her boyfriend's actions, the firm reminder that condoms are necessary to prevent the spread of STDs—had been delivered casually but with an authority that I begin to understand I needed to truly believe. I am grown up now, as Carrie will someday be, and now seems as good a time as any to stop apologizing. I know that there are patients with whom I cannot so immediately relate and from whom I have to quell the instinct to shy away, the sullen girls from bad neighborhoods who fall asleep at night despite the gunshots and the voices raised in anger and the shattering of glass. These girls (and boys) inhabit a world filled with so many dangers that unsafe sex seems to them to be the safest thing of all. And though it had seemed kinder (and infinitely easier) at times not to challenge their choices, I realize as I am saying goodbye to Carrie that this would be no different from deciding that I don't really care.

The first patient who I yell at is named Latreese.

She comes in to have a urine test for chlamydia to make sure that the antibiotics she was prescribed when she tested positive have cleared the infection. There is no reason for the antibiotics not to work, and testing her again is the same as saying that we do not trust her to have taken them and do not trust that she has refrained from having unprotected sex with the same partner who gave her the infection in the first place. If Latreese had been a different person, if she had been one of those girls whose mothers wore sweater sets and gave afternoon teas, it is likely she would have been counted on to follow instructions. But she is poor and she is black, so she had been asked to come back to clinic to be tested again. There was a time I would have been indignant at this distinction, but almost a year into my training I have learned that there are some stereotypes that are perpetuated because they are all too often true.

I have never met Latreese before and she has already peed in the cup by the time I walk into her exam room. In this way, too, she is being treated as second class. She is not seeing a doctor who has seen her before, who can rush things along and finish the visit quickly and send her on her way. That sort of respect should be given to everyone, but it is not possible in these clinics where we residents rotate because we only work in any one place for a few weeks at a time. It is likely that Latreese is unaware of this distinction, does not know that there are doctors in offices just down the street who only accept private insurance and who personally see each of their own patients every time one of them walks through the door. She does not know that there are doctors who are available by phone after hours or who would come by to see her if she were ever in the hospital, because that is the right thing to do. Latreese only knows that doctors' offices are crowded and that the wait is most often as long as it is annoying. It is why she did not come to be seen at all between the ages of fifteen and eighteen and why it was only after the discharge became so bad that she needed to wear a sanitary napkin during the night to keep it from soaking through her underpants that she finally came in for an exam.

I learn all this from her computerized records before my afternoon clinic session begins. I do not read everything because my time is limited and because there is a good chance that she will not show. But here she is, and for once I do not have anyone waiting, so I can take whatever time we need to talk.

"How have things been going?" I ask after the first introductions.

She shrugs; it is what all teenagers do best. "Fine, I guess."

"Do you know why you're here today?"

She crosses and then uncrosses slim legs encased in skintight denim. The gold bangles on her left wrist make a delicate rustling sound as they strike up against each other.

"Sure. To make sure that the infection is gone."

I nod in encouragement.

"Good. And do you know the name of the infection that you had?"

"It was an STD."

I nod again and tell her, "You're absolutely right. It's called chlamydia. I know it's kind of a funny word, but it's important to remember the name in case you ever needed to talk with a doctor who doesn't have access to your records."

The look she gives me says "whatever," but she does not speak.

"Do you know how you got the infection?"

"You get it from having sex."

This is, strictly speaking, true, but it is not the answer to the question I actually asked. Her sentence could have been taken from an informational leaflet or quoted from a health teacher at her school. The question I asked her was one of responsibility and it was one that she chose to dodge.

"Who were you having sex with?" I ask her.

"My boyfriend," she tells me as if I should have known.

"How long have the two of you been sleeping together?" I ask to get some sense of the timeline.

"About a year."

"And did you have sex with anyone else while the two of you were together?"

"No."

From her records I know that she had a negative urine screen for both gonorrhea and chlamydia at a visit not long after she turned nineteen. That was three months before her symptoms began and about four months after she and her boyfriend started having sex.

So I say, just to be sure we are clear, "You know that the infection came from him then."

"Yes," and she says this almost proudly, "I told him that if he ever did anything like that again, then he wouldn't get another chance."

She does not use the word *cheat*, does not acknowledge the obvious betrayal. Still I am relieved to find that she has set some sort of boundaries even if I am uncertain about where exactly she has decided to lay down this line.

"You know that if he did do something like that again that he might not just give you chlamydia, which is something we can treat. He could give you HIV. You could get AIDS if you are not using condoms."

"He wouldn't do that."

"He might not know that he is doing it."

She lifts one arm and the bracelets slide down the thin wrist. She opens and closes her cell phone and puts it back into her bag.

"Has he been treated for the chlamydia?"

"Yes."

"And you're sure that you've used condoms all the time before you were both treated?"

"Oh, we're not having sex now."

It is unlikely that this is some personal journey toward greater purity and I am suspicious of the casual tone that she has adopted. It is clear that she would like me to believe that this is a matter of no consequence. People have sex all the time. Why shouldn't they also, on occasion and for a time, not do so instead?

"Is there a reason that you stopped?"

If she is having pain and does not want to have intercourse, then that is important to find out.

"He got sent away."

I am not entirely sure that I am down with the vernacular, but I take a chance and say, "How long will he be in jail for?"

"I think for six more months."

"And the two of you are still together? You're sticking by him?"

She nods. This is the point at which I would too often have left it. My own boyfriends were not the sort that got sent to prison. They cheated, they lied, and they manipulated, but they did not, as far as I knew, end up behind bars. So I would not usually have pushed when faced with such an obvious departure from what I found familiar. But I had made a promise, to myself and to Latreese, and it was one I was determined to at least try to keep.

"That must be hard," I acknowledge, because it must be even if I think she is probably better off on her own.

It is an uncomfortable conversation to be having, but I ask the question anyway.

"What did he do to get arrested?"

"You know how it is when you're on probation. You can't do anything wrong at all."

"What did he do this time?" I ask firmly to make it clear that I will not let this go.

"He was with a girlfriend of mine when they were going out. We broke up for a little while and he went out with her. She called the police on him."

She would like me to believe that whatever caused her boyfriend to be in jail was this friend's fault and not his own.

"Did he hit her?"

She shakes her head in the affirmative instead of saying it out loud.

"That's not okay!" I yell, somewhat startled by the volume of my voice.

I know that I am judging her by saying this, for taking him back when he begged her to, for not turning him away, and I hope that she will tolerate this intrusion for the kindness it is meant to be, that I am angry for her and not at her, that there is a distinction between the two. There is the chance that she will simply shut the conversation down, but it is a risk I have to take.

"He would never hurt me."

I am absolutely sure this is untrue, but I also know I have no way of convincing her.

"That doesn't really matter," I say instead. "He shouldn't ever hurt anyone."

We look at each other while Latreese fidgets with her bedazzled bag and bracelet. Though I do not really feel as bold as the girl before me, I do not look away.

In the end it does not really matter that my private and very small transformation has taken place. Latreese has been cleared of her chlamydia and will either wait around to be with this particular boyfriend or will decide that she has better things to do. I do not kid myself that the look we shared, only a few seconds really, held any importance for her. She will not look back on that moment when the next time it is her face that his fist slams into; she will not have gained from one short doctor's visit the strength needed to walk away. That strength is there inside her already, or else it is not. I, however, will look back on that visit more than once, will remember what it felt like to yell. And I will be grateful to Latreese for helping me grow up, even if I could not help her do the same.

I have much more hope for Allison, thirteen years old and in the hospital after having a swollen knee tapped downstairs in the ER. During questioning she must have admitted that she was having sex, although when I talk to her after she is sent up to the floor, I find that she has only actually had intercourse three times. She did not use condoms. Although the fluid that they took from her red and painful knee does not appear to be grossly infected, it is not possible to rule out gonorrhea until the culture results come back. She is in the hospital on IV antibiotics until this happens, and her mother is fit to be tied.

"I need to find a new doctor for her," her mother says.

"It might be a good idea for her to see an adolescent doc," I agree. "That way, when it's time for her to have a gyn exam, they can just do it there. She wouldn't have to go someplace separate."

"What sort of exam?" Allison asks.

There is no way she has gonorrhea from having sex with her fourteen-year-old boyfriend who was also a virgin. But whoever saw her down in the ER was right that they could not be absolutely sure.

"After women start having sex, they need to have regular exams of their cervix, the bottom part of the uterus, and so we use a speculum to help us take a look."

I explain what a speculum looks like and how it is inserted.

"That's disgusting. I don't want that inside me."

I do not think before I say, "It's a lot cleaner than some of the other things you've been putting in."

It is the sort of comment I could probably get fired for, and for a fraction of a second I feel as if I may actually vomit. I do not have much time to worry, though, because Allison's mother puts one fist into the air and shakes it.

"Thank you! That's what I'm talking about," she exclaims, and I know that Allison, embarrassed though she is right now, will probably be all right.

Before letting Latreese leave, I find our supervising doctor in the back conference room and summarize all that has been said. Dr. Prewitt pokes her head into the exam room just to meet the patient, but there is nothing else really to do. Latreese's urine test results will be called in to her when they are available. I have already printed her refills for her birth control in case she runs out before she comes back to the clinic again.

Dr. Prewitt is near retirement and she has maintained her hair a saucy and shocking red.

"It's so hard for girls these days," she says, her voice infused with what I interpret as regret.

"She's been dealt a bum hand," I tell her in agreement and try to formulate a way to ask her how she manages to maintain the energy needed to face these sorts of girls.

But instead she tells me, "No, it's all girls. It's you as well. I really thought it would be easier for your generation."

She tells me that she has recently started dating again after the death of her husband, and whenever she is chatted up by some dashing gentleman, things go well until he finds out that she is a professor at the medical school and then he promptly finds a poorly scripted reason to flee.

"Most men are not ready to handle a strong woman."

I tell her that I know this is true.

"You girls have the hardest time of all. You're smart; you're doctors. I'm sure they get scared away."

"I do think it's hard for the people who are still single to find any time to meet new people at all."

"What does your husband do?" she asks me, eyes bobbing down to my wedding ring.

I tell her that he is a physicist.

"Another brain. Well, I hope you found a good one."

I do not answer. Instead, I smile, indicating that I realize—especially when compared to Latreese—just how lucky I am. I love my husband. I know that he loves me. I do not have to worry that he will hit me when he is angry or even when he is not.

Still, no relationship is perfect, and this varies only in degree. It was not my job to fix Latreese's relationship or anyone else's but my own. Still it was, and would be for as long as teenagers continue to do foolish things, my job to listen. And when I had finished listening, it would be my job to tell them what I thought even if it was not something they wanted to hear.

How to Exit Stage Right

After seventy nights during that first year spent on call in the hospital (fumbling through paperwork, answering pages, and writing orders as new children arrive on the floor), I still reach a point of exhaustion at three or four a.m. that is difficult to push through. I am not used to it, as they said I would be. I have not settled into a state of graceful acceptance and instead still frequently resent the unattended weddings and birthdays, the missed connections with friends passing through town for a weekend when I am invariably on call. I still tack up my schedule each month and concentrate on not panicking. I still cross each calendar day off with a red marker after it has been endured. Then, when on the eve of my junior year I lie awake in my bed for the full eight hours I had expected to be able to sleep in preparation for the next thirty hours of call that I have ahead, I realize that they had also lied when they said internship would be the hardest thing I would ever do.

The medical surgical intensive care unit (MSICU) is on the seventh floor and it is enormous. Despite the busy cardiac ICU one floor above and the Intermediate Care Program one floor up again, where many of the children are just as sick as those in ICUs elsewhere, the MSICU has recently expanded to accommodate the growing need for critical care services for a population of chronically ill children who are living for longer than they ever have before. It is a place of near misses, where death is a thing that is rarely overcome but at best held precariously at bay.

It is here that I meet Max. He is seventeen and was diagnosed with acute lymphoblastic leukemia (ALL) more than five years ago. His last set of treatments included a second bone marrow transplant that seems to have finally taken the leukemia away. He is awake for only a handful of hours when he first arrives from the outside hospital where, in the ER there and during transport, he had been started on both dopamine and norepinephrine to keep his blood pressure from continuing to fall. At the very same time that Max reaches the unit, an infant is returning to the floor after a long and not terribly successful surgery to remove the tumor sitting at the bottom of her brain. Unlike Max's, her blood pressure is too high and a worrying sign that her intracranial pressure might be rising enough to push parts of her brain down into the hole that the spinal cord passes through. Orders must be written, management plans must be made, and the more than a dozen other very sick patients for whom I am primarily responsible cannot be entirely neglected as I try to triage the work that must be done.

This is why I speak to Max only in passing as I complete my physical exam. I confirm the story that he awoke today with shortness of breath that has been getting increasingly more severe. As he gasps, his mouth open wide, I do not make him wade through his past medical history because there is not enough air in his lungs to tell me even a small part of what he has suffered. In any case, I have already been handed a detailed written summary of Max's history by the oncology fellow who is on call overnight and I have been briefed by the transport team about all that has happened while they were en route. Any gaps in the story can be filled in once Max's parents arrive.

I lightly rest my stethoscope over Max's heart just to the right of the central venous access port that had been surgically implanted beneath his skin to deliver chemotherapy and is now being used to run the infusions that keep his blood pressure just high enough to maintain the circulation to his body and then back to his heart. The skin covering the thin chest wall is sallow. As he struggles to catch his breath, each rib is starkly visible, making his thinness all the more pronounced. Like his upper body, the legs that emerge from beneath the faded hospital gown are without fat and decorated with liver spots. His is the body of an old man made complete by his baldness. It is only his face that seems preserved—childlike even—although this, too, is as much a falsehood as his otherwise aged form, the soft flesh filling out each of his cheeks more likely a side effect of treatment with steroids than a visage that has been left miraculously unchanged. Still the contrast is remarkable and makes his bravery unexpected, coming as it does from such a shrunken figure with the soft features of a boy. He is heartbreakingly polite as I tell him that we are giving him oxygen to make it easier for him to breathe, to get him feeling better, while we fix this thing that has gone wrong.

I am reassuring, although in reality I have no clear idea what lies ahead. Max would be given whatever support he needed to breathe, with oxygen or positive pressure through a mask or even a breathing tube if it progressed to that. The other things that are needed to keep a person alive, fluids and nutrition, could be given intravenously until his breathing troubles resolved. These are not minor interventions, but neither are they wholly outside the realm of the routine here in the ICU where—of all places in the hospital—you might begin to believe that miracles can occur. All these things together would be used to plot a course that moved slowly to the eventual goal of sending Max home again.

"Meticulous management," our attending Dr. Stegg would say each morning before rounds and during our review of Max's most recent chest X-ray. "That's how we're going to get Max through this alive."

It was not so much a warning as a promise, this daily recitation so like the murmured words of prophets in a bustling town square spoken to give the people hope. It never occurred to me that I could not believe him, that Max's story would ever end any other way.

It certainly would not be an easy fix. Each day's films showed the fluffy opacities that uniformly filled Max's lungs and that were evidence both of his current acute respiratory distress syndrome (ARDS) and his past battle with pulmonary aspergillosis, a fungal infection that had almost killed him several months before when all of the airspaces that should be dark on the film had precipitously filled with blood.

Dr. Stegg turns his gaze from this film or another like it and looks at me.

"How are we going to get through rounds?"

And I answer as I have been trained to, "Like a knife through butter."

"That's right," he nods and says in a caricature of himself reminiscent of *Saturday Night Live*, "Like a knife through buddah."

With this daily encouragement to galvanize us, we walk around to each of the patient rooms and either I or Leisha, my fellow junior on this team, present the overnight events. We touch base with the nurses. We make our plan for the day. We save Max for last always and page the oncology team before we begin so that they can be there to hear our assessment. I present using a printout of Max's morning vitals and his most recent labs. The data spills off the usual double-sided page and onto a second, in addition to which I have copied out the results of each of his blood gases, numbers that represent the success with which he is being oxygenated and ventilated, which are sent to the lab at intervals of every few hours when he is stable and even more frequently when he is not. I speak quickly, trying not to lapse into commentary as I organize the strings of lab values in a way that will highlight the gains and losses in his condition and help us move on to the more important question of what exactly to do.

Each morning I do this before an audience that includes the attending and more than one fellow, one or two ICU residents, three nurses, two respiratory therapists, three or four members of the oncology consult service, and one or both of Max's parents. When I have presented the numbers and reviewed a list of medications that includes antibiotics and antifungals for an infection that we know is there but remain unable to isolate, insulin to manage Max's blood sugar, sedatives to keep him comfortable, diuretics to help take the fluid out of his lungs, and chemotherapeutic agents to prevent any remaining leukemic cells from proliferating again, I begin to outline my management plan for the day.

Max himself is not a part of these discussions, not because the number of people involved would not fit into his room, although they probably wouldn't, but because on his second day in the hospital his respiratory distress became so severe that it was necessary to use a ventilator to help him breathe. Shortly after this, the traditional ventilator is switched out for a model that delivers small and very frequent breaths to minimize repeated stretching of the lungs and to prevent as much as possible the inflammation and fluid collection that this stretching would provoke. To allow the ventilator to work at all, Max must be sedated heavily and his muscles paralyzed, which requires ever-increasing doses of opiates. If you squeeze his hand, he does not squeeze back. He is given earplugs to dampen the continuous jetting of the high-frequency ventilator that is like a wash cycle forever in its final spin, but there is no way of telling what he actually hears.

His parents have been through this before, although it has never been quite so bad. His mother, who quit her job when he was first diagnosed, is the one who keeps watch during the day. They split up the nighttime shifts so that one of them is at home in time to have dinner with their two younger girls while the other sleeps in the hospital with Max. It is through his parents that I come to know him. He is at once a boy with cancer, a dissatisfied teenager, and a lovely and caring young man who worries about college and how to find a life where being a patient does not define him. I do not remember any of the things that Max said to me on that first day when he was awake, but I know from his father that despite all the days of school he has missed, he has fallen only a few classes behind his grade. He had been eager to leave the hospital during his last hospitalization in order to finish his junior year by summer school so that he could be a senior at the same time as his friends.

A few weeks into his hospital stay, there is a night when his abdomen becomes swollen and hard, and it looks like Max might die. The general surgeons are consulted because of the concern that he might have a perforation somewhere in his GI system, but it is only a formality. If this is really the case, there is nothing they can do. Almost exactly one year before this, the same thing had happened to Connor—the first patient I ever cared for—and for the same reasons the surgeons had refused to intervene. An operation would surely kill Max and there is no reason to take that risk.

"What a shame," the surgical resident says when he comes to evaluate Max. "He certainly doesn't deserve one more problem on top of all those he's already got."

And the ICU fellow, a small perky girl from whom I never expected to hear such words of doom, replies, "He had a mortality rate of more than 90 percent the minute that he rolled through our door."

The surgeon looked in at Max for just a moment more and then he turned away.

"Well, if he really has perforated somewhere, then that brings his survival down to nil."

I realize finally how the odds are so badly stacked against him. Until this point, I had always believed that it was a matter of careful finesse and patience but that Max—and the numbers I read out in morning rounds—would eventually come out all right. It feels almost like betrayal that they are betting so harshly against him. At the same time, I am embarrassed for having been so naive as to think that we would eventually all sail through this together. If I had expected catastrophe, if I had prepared for carnage, would I have picked up on some sign that might have been there all the time? And because it happened so precipitously, both the change in Max's condition and my understanding of it, I feel responsible but also scared.

Not all children are meant to be saved. I learned this in the NICU and I learned it again now, in the clean and brightly lit halls of the MSICU, behind the sliding glass doors of which lay the near-drownings, the NICU graduates, and the transfers from the oncology floor. The beds and cribs in each of these spaces were as carefully arranged as places of worship, festooned with IV poles and oxygen monitors instead of gilded statues or baptismal fonts. These rooms were not shrines, not exactly, but they contained within them much the same idea, despite the differences in appearance, despite the absence of cool stone and bare feet and shallow pools with floating blossoms exploding slowly as their color deepens into brilliance and then fades away.

The rooms contained at their center the small crumpled body of an infant dragged too late from the water and now in a perpetual slumber interrupted only by fits of sweaty frenzy that are not dreams or nightmares but only the physical manifestation of fear in the release of epinephrine triggered by a brain that was too long deprived of oxygen. Or they contained the man-child who has never walked or sat or opened his eyes in the whole of his twenty-one years of life, who has a trach collar situated just at the base of his throat through which the machine next to him delivers one breath and then another, and a tube that runs directly into his stomach through which he receives feeds. Or the room contains the child with terminal cancer, who has undergone all of the treatments—both standard and experimental—and for whom all the possible treatments failed.

There is one such child who comes to us from one floor below after her first unexplained seizure and the subsequent MRI that shows the bleeding inside her head. I do not know Sammy, but I have met her father, who comes to stand outside the room during each morning's rounds, a slight Eastern European man with a long scar across his left cheek. What I know about Sammy is what I was told in sign-out from Leisha, an outline only, what I need to be aware of in case of emergencies overnight. I know her medications. I know the plan the neurologists have made with her family for managing her seizures and that there was a long meeting with both parents that very afternoon. It is not everything; it is not the color of her eyes or the way her lips are pressed together when she smiles, but it should be enough.

Before this, when she was still at home and able to play despite having marrow and blood composed almost entirely of leukemic blasts, her doctors had said, "What is it that she wants more than anything else?"

And her parents, for whom English words seemed to hold a bitter taste even after so many years in this country and from whose lips even vowels seemed angry and hard, had said, "She keeps asking to go to Disney World."

"Do you think you can take her?"

"Yes," they had nodded. "But we would like to make it a Christmas present. We will go in December."

Then the oncologist who knew them best, who had been there in the beginning when Sammy was just four and she was a resident and later a fellow, who had been there at the bedside when the family first learned her diagnosis six years earlier, said to them, "You need to go now," even though she knew that they would not listen.

They did not go. Two months later, Sammy is in the hospital for the last time.

The cells in her blood are all cancer and she does not have enough platelets to form a good clot at the site of the small tears that even healthy blood vessels sustain every day. This is the reason for the blood in her brain and the subsequent seizures and the frequent transfusions of red cells and platelets that have since been pumped into her arm. It is the reason that her family has been offered the comfort room down on the oncology ward where they would have privacy and space enough for family and friends to visit and sit and for both parents to sleep comfortably each night. It is a space for farewells that is given only to those children and parents who have stopped all the medicines, who have agreed to forego all "heroic measures" of any kind, and who are truly saying goodbye.

Sammy had stayed there before. The comfort room was comfortable, was more homey and spacious than any of the other rooms they might have been offered, so they requested it whenever Sammy fell ill. Then there had been flowers and balloons and the constant traffic of cousins and neighbors. There had been, in one tiny corner of a hospital that was action and movement, peace of a kind. It was in this peace that Sammy had drifted, through light and darkness, through a year's worth of days, and she had moved closer to dying, but in the final approach her parents had always said, "Please." It was with a single word that the contract was always broken, for it is a promise that no parent can be expected to make without pain, the promise to let go, so the blade of the laryngoscope had been flipped open, the tiny light that shines down the back of the throat had gone on, and the doctor who was on call would slip the tube past the glistening curve of Sammy's vocal cords and use a bag to deliver an artificial gust of air.

Finally, they were told no. They were reminded in no uncertain terms that a DNR order, required to be admitted to that room, would be binding if they were not there to object when Sammy started going downhill. If Sammy stopped breathing when they were not right there beside her, then she would be let go. So they refused to sign the order that said "Do Not Resuscitate" because it was not an order in which they believed. Sammy, at the start of this admission, had been placed in an ordinary room just like the one beside it, a room that was adequate but was not special and about which her parents would frequently complain. Her parents took out their anger at this situation and at all of the things that could have been different but weren't, so a visit with Sammy was an ordeal that was not to be entered into without preparing for the onslaught that was to come.

I am called to Sammy's room not long after the seizures first begin and she has been transferred to the unit upon the recommendation of the neurology team. It is the first of two ICU stays during this last hospitalization. In these early days, Sammy is still awake, she is eating and drinking. But she is cranky, and there are times that she yells at her parents and there are times that she refuses to speak and then begins to cry. She is ten and she is trapped—in this hospital room and in a body that will not last her long enough to ride the Thunder Mountain Railroad or climb into the massive and sprawling tree house that the Robinsons had built after their ship had run afoul in the storm.

It is six in the morning and I have not slept for more than twenty-four hours. I am wrestling with a printer that should be spitting out the pages of patient information each of my fellow residents will need for rounds. The Spectralink phone in my scrubs pocket rings as it has done every five or ten minutes since this shift began, and Sammy's nurse, Charmaine, curtly informs me that Sammy's mother had refused the dose of her antiseizure medicine that she was meant to receive at three. She is telling me three hours late, is tidying things up now before the end of her shift so that she can sign off to whoever comes in to relieve her. I know that all she wants from me is to acknowledge this message so that she can move on to the next check box in the pile of paperwork she must have before her. Sammy's mother has the right to refuse whatever medicines she wants because her daughter is dying, her daughter cannot be saved, and while for an otherwise healthy girl this decision could be overridden in the interests of her safety, for Sammy there will be no real difference in outcome if she is given the medicine or if she is not. Still, Sammy has been brought to the ICU so that she can be monitored, closely and with a whole bank of sensors, while the antiseizure medicine runs in. She has been brought to the ICU because of the side effects of this medicine even more than the seizures, so it is no small thing for her mother to choose now to say no.

I ask Charmaine the reason for this refusal and her answer is a mixed-up explanation of how the medicine (or so Sammy's mother believes) is the reason that the girl sometimes yells and sometimes cries and is not as cheerful as her mother wishes her to be. I am already moving while the nurse continues this rambling recitation, repeating many of the things that had been discussed during the hour-long meeting with the neurologists late into the previous afternoon.

I introduce myself as Charmaine and I walk into the room where Sammy's mother sits beside her daughter and I say, "I'm told that you don't feel comfortable giving Sammy the medicine that we're using to control her seizures."

Her mother shakes her head, her thin, straight hair sweeping across her shoulders: "I do not like that medicine. It makes her face go dark."

It is a phrase she has used before to describe this change in Sammy's mood, but neither the oncologists who know Sammy nor the neurologists who are frequently called to link personality changes to underlying organic causes are concerned that Sammy is behaving this way. She is dying, even if her parents refuse to admit this, and she has every reason to be upset.

"It was my understanding that you had met with the neurologists for quite some time yesterday and that you had decided together that giving Sammy this medicine was the best thing for her."

"I told them that I did not like the medicine."

"But she got this medicine all day yesterday and last night," I remind her, "and you didn't object then."

"Her face goes dark and I told the neurologists. I didn't like them. They didn't listen. I want a different medicine."

"It's possible that there may be another medicine that we could use to treat Sammy's seizures, but I'm not a neurologist and so I'm not the right person to make that decision. If we give her this morning's dose now, then the neurologists can meet with you later today and you can discuss your concerns with them."

"When could they come?"

I am acutely aware that it is never a good idea to make promises that it will be up to someone else to keep.

"I'm not sure exactly. The day team will probably not be in until seven, but most likely closer to eight."

"I can wait until seven."

"I can't be sure that they would be available to come straight here first thing this morning. They may have rounds to do."

Charmaine, who had been hovering in the doorway, chooses this moment to speak: "There's a neurologist in the hospital twenty-four hours a day. This is one of the best children's hospitals in the country. They should come right now."

This is an incredibly inappropriate comment and I am too shocked in that moment to be angry. There is one neurology resident in the whole hospital to manage consults in the ER and on the floor. Alone, he or she must sort out the migraines from the brain tumors, respond quickly in case of a code for a seizure that cannot be controlled. It is not this poor young doctor's job to walk into the middle of a conflict that apparently had not been resolved despite more than two hours of debate. It is also not an appropriate message for Sammy's mother to hear, that in this desperate situation where she has no control over the cancer that has taken such a strong hold over her daughter that she can control those people around her, that she can wake up scared and alone in a hospital room and call whatever consult service she wants to speak with her right away.

I had never met Charmaine before she called me, so it is difficult to challenge, to turn to her and say, "The person who is on call is here to take care of emergencies. This isn't an emergency."

It is clear that Charmaine is upset so I cut her off as she prepares to speak and turn to Sammy's mother instead.

"You certainly have the right to refuse the medication. If you don't want her to have it, then we won't give it to her. But I need to hear you tell me that you understand that this medicine is being used to prevent Sammy from having another seizure and that without the medicine it's possible that she could seize."

This is what Charmaine had been trying to pass off to me over the phone, this responsibility for the things that might happen. But it was not mine to take. I did not know Sammy; I did not know the number of bone marrow transplants she had been given or the different rounds of chemotherapy she had undergone. I knew only those things I had to know in order to get her safely through the night, and the fosphenytoin that she was meant to be given—the medication she had missed for an unforgivable amount of time after the dose had been due—was integral to that plan. It would not save her life, so I was not in a position to force it on her, but neither did I believe she should be treated as if medicines or procedures or surgeries were desserts from a pastry kitchen, to be picked over and considered, from which her family was free to choose depending on their mood.

Sammy's mother says again, "The neurologists didn't listen when I said that I did not like this drug."

I am kneeling before her so that my eyes are level with her own and I know that I am too close, but I do not back away.

"If you don't want us to give her the medicine, then I need you to tell me that you understand that without it she could have a seizure."

She snaps with a good deal of venom: "I don't like the way you are talking to me."

I want nothing more in that moment than to leave the room, but I stay. I do not tell her that I, too, have things that I do not like, that I wish I could change, things that I long to have control over, but that despite the years of training and studying, I am often left as helpless as she is. Rather I remain as I am, kneeling on the hard tiles, waiting for her to accept responsibility for the decision that she has made.

"I need you to tell me that you understand."

The woman spits the words out, "I understand," and I am free to go.

I stand and turn despite the pain as the blood returns to my legs. I do not stop when Charmaine, persistent despite my earlier rebuttal, calls after me, "You'll page the neurologist right away?"

"I'll page the neurologist," I reply.

I leave the room and return to the bank of computers where my fellow residents are now seated. They are newly arrived and reviewing the blood gases and fluid balances from overnight, the stack of printouts I had abandoned when Charmaine called, which one of them retrieved and sorted into piles.

"Are you ready to sign out?" Leisha asks me.

"I just need to do one quick thing first."

I am aware that there had been an element of cruelty in the exchange that just took place and I am not at all sure that I have handled it well. It would have been far easier not to have pressed, easier for Sammy's mother, for Charmaine, easier for me. But it was not my job to let changes in Sammy's treatment pass by unnoticed, even out of kindness. It was not Sammy's mother who was my patient, it was Sammy, and although each child's parents and their wishes are important, they cannot be allowed to become more important than the child herself.

It is only just becoming the day shift and I page the neurology resident who is coming on to ask that her team come by to speak again with the family as soon as they conveniently can. While she acknowledges the difficulty of the situation, she is also dismissive, and it is clear that she will not come right away. I begin to feel better, that I have not grossly misjudged the situation, the way things should be expected to work.

Later, after I have signed out the overnight events to Leisha and the other junior residents, I walk around to examine my own charges and to make sure that I have the most up-to-date settings on their ventilators and sedative drip rates. Outside Sammy's room, I see Charmaine speaking with the charge nurse and I know that their discussion is about me. I have all at once the urge to turn and avoid them and also to force a confrontation of some sort, for now I feel the anger that before I had been too shocked to register. I have never been one for picking fights. Months earlier, I would never have sought out Charmaine to tell her that I thought she had erred, that she had broken ranks by offering up something on my behalf (the on-call neurologist) to Sammy's mother that she was not in a position to give.

I approach Charmaine and the charge nurse and tell them what I had already predicted: "The neurology team will come back and see the family this morning, but they can't come right away."

"You shouldn't have told her that Sammy could seize without the medication," the charge nurse says to me. "Now we all better hope that she doesn't have a seizure, because then we're responsible. You shouldn't have put the idea into her head."

It is an odd moment, for I had been under the impression that we would all be responsible no matter where fingers were pointing, no matter what accusations might be made. I had also been under the impression that being honest with families, making sure that they are informed, is a fairly important part of the way this system should work. I should have told them this without a pause, forcefully and without stumbling over the edges of my words, and I do tell them later, in my head, many times over, but in that second I falter.

Instead, all that I can muster is, "It would be worse if Sammy had a seizure and no one had ever warned her that's what could happen."

I say this and I see that they do not agree, but I realize then that I do not have the time or the energy to argue further. I leave to check on a previously healthy teenage boy who was inexplicably septic and who had come in the night before, knowing that the discussion will continue in my absence. Then I round, and in the hours that we walk the halls discussing patients, the tension surrounding Sammy's management somehow shrinks and comes into perspective, until it is merely one of many check boxes on a list that contains two dozen names aside from hers.

I am not there when Sammy dies, but in sensing so strongly that it is coming, I yearn for it in a way. Death is the stray bullet; it is the masked horseman; it is the thing against which you concentrate all of your efforts and for which you can never prepare. It is also, in this hospital for children, where octogenarians do not lie beneath each set of bedsheets mumbling toothlessly over their rosary beads, relatively rare. But death is concentrated in the ICU, where those recovering from difficult surgeries or whose blood pressures have begun to run dangerously low are whisked away to be patched up if not entirely repaired, or, at the very least, made as comfortable as possible when nothing more can be done.

When Sammy leaves the ICU, stable enough to return to the oncology floor, I have been a doctor for just over a year and I have never seen a child die. I have cared for those who eventually would, but I have not stood beside a mother and seen what happens when the chest finally ceases its irregular and asynchronous rise and fall. Then, one night not long after Sammy leaves us to go back downstairs, while Max continues to require ever-increasing doses of morphine and pentobarbital to keep him calm and asleep, I am on call when an eleven-day-old infant girl dies.

She had been born with a hole in her diaphragm, with almost no separation between the spaces inside that were meant to be divided into her abdomen and chest. Because of this hole, her intestines had herniated, had slithered upward to envelop her heart, leaving her delicate lungs without enough volume to expand with each liquid breath as she was growing inside. For some of these children, the hole is a small one, the herniation of bowel not too severe. The lungs are underdeveloped but functional, and with multiple surgeries the contents of the infant's abdomen can be rearranged so that they stay where they are meant to stay. But Baby Girl Bristlethwait is not one of those children. She had been born by C-section in an operating room just a few floors below; normally the obstetricians would deliver the child in the adult hospital just next door, and expect the critical care staff to rush the incubator across the bridge between the two buildings, but Baby Girl Bristlethwait would in all likelihood not have survived the journey.

Her diaphragmatic hernia is quite severe. Since her arrival, she had been maintained on a specialized high-frequency ventilator to give her still-fragile lungs the most minuscule breaths possible in order to keep her alive. She had also (because of a deep cleft in her lip) been screened for and diagnosed with a rare syndrome associated with this condition, which would mean further serious medical problems even if she were able to survive. That night, my senior resident and I are preparing to midnight round with the team when the first-year fellow asks if we can wait. He tells us that he just needs a few minutes to withdraw care from Baby Girl Bristlethwait. Her parents have just this evening decided, upon the advice of the surgeons and geneticists, to let her go. It is the life of this couple's brand-new baby, but it is also a lesson I need to see, so I ask if I can come.

Baby Girl Bristlethwait is on a radiant warmer open on all sides with heat coming down from above to compensate for the losses from her small naked form. There are lines attached to her that read her temperature and heart rate and would (were she not on the high-frequency ventilator) register each breath that she takes. She is not in a room but rather an open bay with space enough for four different patients, although on this particular night it holds only three. One of these is an infant girl just three days younger than Baby Girl Bristlethwait with a diaphragmatic hernia that will be relatively easy to repair. The families of these two daughters are separated only by a series of hanging curtains that seem somehow to have been designed to always leave a gap of six inches or so on one end or the other, so they offer at all times to those on the opposite side a glimpse of the scenes taking place just behind.

The fellow introduces himself again to the family and then says my name with a brief gesture toward me. I stay back as he describes what will happen when the ventilator is turned off and the endotracheal tube is pulled out; he explains that she will likely continue to breathe, shallowly and without great effect, and that gradually the lack of oxygen will cause her pulse to slow until her heart comes to a stop. The IVs will be left in, since that is what her parents had said they wanted so that she can continue to receive medicine to make her more comfortable.

Baby Girl Bristlethwait's father is sitting directly at the foot of the warmer with his head slightly bowed. He does not turn to look at the fellow, who moves quietly around the monitors and tubes, but keeps his eyes low. He is not a small man, but he seems dwarfed somehow by the low-backed chair into which he has folded himself, his hunched shoulders, dark neck, and orb of black curly hair a silhouette that remains stationary throughout the whole event.

"You can hold her if you would like," the fellow says, looking first at the statue of her father and then at her young mother, possibly even a teenager, who is wearing red sweatpants and a man's thin white undershirt, the fabric of which stretches across the still-full expanse of her abdomen. She is perched precariously on a high stool several feet from where the infant's father is seated and gives the distinct impression that at any moment she might fall.

The woman shakes her head and then nods toward her partner, who has not responded at all to the fellow's words.

"Let him take her."

The fellow then moves the baby, slowly as she is still attached to the ventilator, and places her on a pillow that has been set across her father's lap. The head and the shoulders of this man remain immobile, but he does move one finger to rest in the curve of her tiny palm. The fellow leans over the pair and gently peels the anchoring tape from the infant's mouth and nose and removes the breathing tube. In the silence there is laughter from one of the neighboring bed spaces. Baby Girl Bristlethwait's mother begins to cry.

The number that represents the oxygen saturation of the infant's blood drops from the high 90s down to 82. The respiratory therapist, a thin young man with a shark's tooth hanging around his neck, busies himself in connecting blue plastic tubing to the maneuverable arm coming down from the ceiling. Misting oxygen begins to billow from the end and he then tries to Velcro the tube onto the pillow upon which Baby Girl Bristlethwait is lying so that the thin fog can blow in the general direction of her little broken face. When the fellow notices this, he puts up one hand in a small gesture of warning and bends forward to move the tube away. After a long stretch of standing idly, the respiratory therapist notices the intrusive clacking of the water condensing on the side of the tubing and turns the knob to shut off the oxygen supply.

It is unbearable. Even though I had asked to come merely as an observer—so that should it ever be my job to oversee such a tragedy, I would know the things that are right to do and say—I cannot stand the cluttered silence.

"Did you give her a name?" I ask her mother.

The woman inhales deeply and noisily past the snot in the back of her throat. I reach for the box of tissues and slide the trash can closer to the stool where she sits.

"We named her Candi. With an 'i'."

It is a wretched name, but I lie without guilt as I say, "What a wonderful choice."

The infant is breathing slowly. Her heart rate, which had been 140, has dropped to 60, the point at which chest compressions would normally be done. I glance at the fellow, who is also watching the monitor. It is a sad scene but not in the way I had imagined it would be. I know that I should not really be here, or that I should stand unobtrusively, moving only to adjust the curtains to maintain whatever semblance of privacy I can for these people. But there is an isolation here for which I was unprepared: the father and his infant daughter, and the mother sitting high above, not touching. It is as if the thing that is happening is happening to each of them alone. As they are making no move whatsoever to comfort each other, I place a hand on Candi's mother's shoulder.

"Does she have any brothers or sisters?" I ask.

The woman nods. Her unwashed hair is lifted by the movement and then sticks to the shoulders of the cheap cotton shirt. "She does. She has a four-year-old sister."

"Did they get to meet?"

The woman takes another tissue from the box in my outstretched hand.

"Yeah. We brought her in so she could see the baby and touch her."

"That's nice that they spent some time together."

Dying is a slow process, even for this infant who had no chance at all to truly live. She stops breathing for long spaces of time while her heart rate idles around 40 and then she begins to breathe again. Each time she does, her lips part, and the gash on the left side widens and gives the impression that it might bleed.

"She's so beautiful," I say, knowing that it is both a falsehood and a truth.

Candi's mother sniffles again and wipes a river of tears from her face.

"Thank you."

Later, when Candi has at last stopped breathing, when her heart has become still, I back slowly away and move sideways out through the curtains, turning to close them carefully behind me. My senior resident is seated still before one of a bank of computers, reviewing the results of a rugby tournament that had happened earlier in the day.

"Are we rounding?" he asks.

"Yes," I tell him. "I think pretty soon."

Death is an obvious answer to the question of what it is about medicine and pediatrics in particular that can make its practice difficult, but death itself is simple. It is a single moment, and a moment, no matter how painful the flash of grief that accompanies it, is easy enough to endure. Death is nothing compared to all the moments that lead up to it and those that follow. It is in this span of time that things may be handled well or badly, that inattentiveness or hunger or selfishness can disrupt the scene. And the guilt that is often felt by doctors looking on is borne not only of the fact that this life in particular could not be saved, although that guilt, too, is certainly keenly felt, but because it is also our responsibility to see to and to orchestrate death itself.

When this month has reached its end, all that is left is to go through the now familiar process of handing off my patient list to my replacement. I have not worked with Vassilios before, but we live only blocks from each other and have occasionally bumped into each other at the supermarket or local burrito joint. He is unflappable and well organized. I know that I will be leaving my patients in excellent hands. When I page him to sign out, it is approaching dinnertime. He is at the park with his son, but he calls back almost immediately. In the spaces between our words, I discern the screams of children, the shrill, short outbursts that are a combination of startled terror and sheer delight. I imagine the creaking of the chains that hold the plastic swings, the soft explosion of sawdust as Velcroed sneakers make their landing, the crunch of gravel beneath the wheels of strollers being pushed toward home.

"Is now an okay time?" I ask, desperately hoping that it is, having begun to taste, now that it has come so close, the freedom that will come with handing over this responsibility, the anticipation and relief at looking forward to the next month of caring for children who (in contrast to those in the ICU) I might be able to help get well enough to actually go home.

"Now is a great time."

"I just e-mailed you the updated discharge summaries and the sign-out. Would it be easier for you to talk with the e-mail in front of you?"

"No," he tells me. "This is fine. I'll read through it when I get home, and I can always call you if I have questions."

"I only have a few kids for you, and only one of them is a long-term player, so it shouldn't be too bad."

This is a sentence of some significance and I linger over it for a moment. I have only just, in the last several days, managed to discharge those rocks (patients who never seem to move closer to leaving no matter the effort exerted in pushing them along the way) whom I had inherited at the beginning of the month or whom I had admitted myself just after the rotation had begun. These were children who would never have more than a few days at a time at home, who pass their time here swinging like the bob of a pendulum between the Franciscans' rehabilitation facility and the ICU. It was a source of some pride that I would not be handing off any of these children to Vassilios. It was also a gift of time each morning (if only just a small collection of minutes) that would not need to be spent gathering vitals or labs on eight patients instead of three, and it was a gift I was happy to be able to give.

I tell Vassilios about the thirteen-year-old girl who got so drunk she needed to be intubated to protect her airway and to ensure that she didn't forget to breathe. I tell him about the neighborhood boy who was found hiding in her shower and how her father was so enraged that he asked us to do a rape kit on her while she was sedated and on the ventilator. I explain how her family had not wanted her to experience the trauma of having the specimens collected after she was awake, despite there not being any evidence at the scene that she was involved sexually with the boy at all. There had been only his terrified presence in the bathroom and the rainbow of colors painted on her nails that one of the EMTs thought was something the kids might be doing now to advertise the number of boys they had kissed or fooled around with, but no one could say for sure. I explain how in the end all of this gossip, which is really what it was, had occurred while she was still asleep and thus unable to defend herself against such accusations of impropriety.

I also tell him about the six-month-old who had been brought in because of a possible seizure. She had a CT of her head that showed fresh bleeding in the front but also bleeding in the back that looked old, and how I had made the call to DSS at four in the morning because there was also a two-year-old in the house. I tell him how, because of the concern that the baby had been shaken, the police had gone on to take her brother in the middle of the night (a frightening event and not a thing I ever thought that I would trigger) and that when she leaves the hospital it will not be to go home. She will join her brother in foster care, because when the ophthalmologists came in the morning to look at the baby's eyes, they found the worst hemorrhages there that any of them had ever seen, blood vessels burst open from the force of her brain smacking repeatedly against the inside of her skull.

Finally, I tell Vassilios about Max. At the end of my month with him, Max is still on a high-frequency ventilator in an attempt to protect his lungs from the trauma of even a normal amount of breathing in and out. His belly is soft, but we have not fed him except through his veins since the night his abdomen had swelled. The labs that keep track of his kidneys look better than they had one week before, but the numbers are still worse than any I had ever seen before. He is being given five different antibiotics and an antifungal to keep whatever infection is still quietly brewing from overwhelming his fragile immune system. He is on three separate sedative medicines to keep him sleeping and still. What I tell Vassilios is that Max is sick. He is sicker than anyone I had ever seen before this rotation began. He is sick, but he is still alive and he has a family who loves him and a life that is waiting on the other side of this now that his cancer is gone.

"Anything else I need to know?"

There is only one other thing, and I say it because it is important and is not necessarily implied.

"Don't let Max die."

I say it out loud in the way that Dr. Stegg, with firm encouragement, often told us that each subtle change in Max's ventilator settings or diuretics was being made so that someday he could go home. I say it as if the words themselves have power, will be amplified and take on substance as they are transmitted by a cell tower and projected into Vassilios's ear. But no words—however earnest, however well intentioned—could ever be enough.

It is three in the morning, about three weeks after I leave the unit, when I check my e-mail during an overnight shift in the ER at the City Hospital and Max has been dead for a little over a day. The e-mail has not been sent to me in particular but to all residents; there had been a similar message about a week before when Sammy, too, had died. I sit rereading the short and unrevealing message on the too-bright computer screen in the lull that sometimes happens in the early morning when a busy emergency room has been emptied out. I sit and I think about where I might be able to go to cry. The night nurses, several yards from where I am and huddled around their own cluster of computers, are munching on a dinner of cheese and apple slices. I am the only resident in the ER. Although it is quiet and I can certainly and justifiably slip away for a moment to visit the soda machine, I cannot be gone for long.

I walk into the hall through the waiting room and past the security desk where a man in a wheelchair is drunkenly demanding cab fare from the officers sitting there, then turn to take the long way around to the nearest vending machines. The halls are dim and I cry, but only a little. I buy a diet soda and move to head back the way I have just come. I had been in to visit not long before when I was last over at Children's, having found myself missing (despite the four weeks of perpetual anxiety it had provoked) the intensity of that floor. At that point Max had been able to transition back to a traditional ventilator, but was slow to wake up after being kept asleep for so long. Even after all of the pain medications and paralytics had been turned off, his eyes remained closed and his fingers (pressed firmly in his father's large hand) were limp and did not exert any pressure of their own.

I am sad for Max, for his parents, but crying feels pointless here where there is no one to see. I would like to cry in the way that children sometimes are able, curled at the foot of my bed with my own mother's hand gently stroking my hair. Then there would be an audience for the inciting injustice; there would be someone to whom I could tell Max's name. But there is no one. In any case, there is nothing I can think of to say that would be nearly enough.

When I return to the ER, the man in the wheelchair is still there at the entrance, sitting quiet now and drifting fitfully toward sleep, his chair pushed into a corner so that he faces the dark night beyond the sliding hospital doors. He smells faintly of urine and cheap aftershave. It is possible that he has a home waiting for him, has loved ones who would miss him if he were gone, but it's hard to tell, looking at the frayed bottoms of his gray sweatpants and the thin bare ankle peeking from the top of one grubby and laceless New Balance shoe. I pause for just a few seconds longer and then walk back into the pediatric ER, past the nearly empty fish tank and the flat-screen television that is playing the menu for the *Surf's Up* DVD on an endless loop, although there is no one there to see.

Two weeks later we have a residents' retreat, the one day out of the year when the hospital services are left in the hands of other doctors, when we can gather as a group to discuss our training program—the things that are working and the things that we need to change. It is a sunny and unexpectedly blistering day in late September, and I catch a ride with one of our chief residents to the venue outside of the city where the day's activities are being held. It is not until after all of the morning's lectures that I see Vassilios. The groups are breaking up from the central meeting room and moving outside for an assortment of trust-building games. He and I are heading toward the same door when we see each other and we stop to let the crowd pass by around us. Vassilios makes a small shrug and shakes his head and then we hug.

"I meant to call you," he says. "I wanted to tell you about Max."

What he tells me is that despite everything we tried to do for him, Max did not ever wake up. After the morphine and the pentobarbital drips had been turned off, he never really stirred. The infection he had had all the while was the same aspergillosis that had nearly killed him months before. His parents, Vassilios reported, said that they were running just on fumes. They decided it was time to stop; it was time to let him go.

Dr. Stegg made most of the arrangements. He met with the nurses to let them know what to expect, to make sure everyone was on board with the plan and there were no last-minute disagreements, no careless words that his parents might remember from that day instead of just remembering spending it with their son.

"Max's dog will be coming in to visit," he told the charge nurse before it happened.

Then there had been a minor fuss. There were questions about infection control, about getting leave from a hospital administrator or the like, about whether guidelines for such an event even existed at all. Dr. Stegg had stood calmly and then cut short this line of inquiry.

"You didn't understand what I said," he said firmly but kindly. "I'm not asking you how I go about getting permission. I'm telling. Max's dog is coming to see him. That's the final word."

Max's dog did come, and he leaped on the bed and licked Max's face around where the endotracheal tube went in. The whole family was together for a little while in that way, the parents and the brother and sisters and their pet, and then they took Max downstairs in an elevator and pushed his bed outside.

In the back of the hospital garden there is an open swath of grass that is well concealed behind ornamental shrubs. From the front, sitting on one of the low stone benches and looking at the fountain of playing otters, you do not know this space is there. It is where they sat with Max, for an hour, before the tube came out, beneath a clear blue sky of early autumn with the sun warming through to the backs of his closed eyelids to turn them bright. It is possible he could feel this change, could still experience this color even if his mind had lost the ability to think *red.* I hope so. I hope also that when the tube came out he was able to take at least one final breath, to wash out the recycled air that had been pushed into him, and to once more smell something that was alive.

Hearing this, I cry, as I had not been able to cry before. The tears are decorous; I do not sob, for I am still at work in a manner of speaking and I have no wish to make a scene. But I do cry, almost with relief, that Vassilios has spoken Max's name out loud and that

I could understand what he had to say. It is with relief also that I think about the manner of his passing, the reverence and solemnity in the final moments but also the not complete absence of joy. It is what we should be able to give to every family, every person who is faced with the departure of a loved one, and it is what we in medicine so rarely still get right. I am grateful to Dr. Stegg for the dog and for the garden and for all the rest he must have done besides. I speak Max's name once more, for good measure, and Vassilios and I step outside and beneath a sky bright with a warm yellow sun that quickly dries the tears as they fall silently onto my cheeks.

Where We Live

"You can't break these kids," our attending Sangeeta tells my fellow resident Venee and me at the halfway point of our junior year. "You can't break them because they're already broken."

We are sitting in the small cramped office in which we do our morning rounds, hidden away instead of standing in the halls outside of patient rooms, both because this process takes so long and because we need privacy for so much of what we have to say. We are discussing an eight-year-old girl named Frances, who is admitted to our service for treatment of a pneumonia that has socked in the lower lobe of one of her lungs. On the surface of things, and compared to the patients I had recently cared for in the ICU, Frances is not all that sick. She should get antibiotics and then she should go home. But she also has seizures, despite the three different antiepileptics that are squirted through her G-tube several times each day. Because she does not speak or sit up or play, these seizures (which cluster in the morning and involve deviation of her eyes to one side and sometimes a subtle but rhythmic twitching of one thumb) are not always apparent. Half of the time, they stop on their own within a matter of minutes, leaving no evidence that anything at all has changed. The other half of the time, they do not stop, so her mother—who also has developmental problems and who still lives with her own parents despite being in her mid-forties—inserts a suppository of a rescue seizure medication called Diastat into Frances's bum. She does this at least once a week and even more often when Frances is sick and her seizure threshold continues to drop.

The seizures themselves are the result of lissencephaly, an abnormal smoothness of the surface of Frances's brain. While she was still a fetus, Frances's brain failed to develop the deep ridges and indentations that are normal. Because of the seizures and the generalized low muscle tone that results from this malformation, it was only by undergoing a tracheostomy that Frances was able to breathe safely. Before this direct opening at the base of her throat was cut, she had suffered recurrent obstruction by her tongue of her upper airway, which had frequently led her to turn blue. Now, even during a seizure, Frances is able to move air easily into her lungs. She breathes shallowly, but it is enough to maintain her oxygen saturation at a reassuring 99 percent. Still, because she cannot cough effectively, phlegm often collects within the trach and needs to be sucked out. She requires constant monitoring, both in the hospital and at home.

Called to her bedside after one of her longer seizures, I am only three hours into a thirty-hour shift when Frances musters the rare effort and actually coughs. The thick yellow sputum that had accumulated in the opening of her tracheostomy button sprays into the air to settle over my face and hair.

"Frances is going to be here for at least a month," Sangeeta tells us as we come out of her room that morning after rounding.

Despite having already cleaned myself up as much and as discreetly as possible, I wipe again at my head with a wet paper towel in a futile attempt to dispel my lingering feeling of disgust.

"Can't we transition her to oral antibiotics once her fever comes down?" Venee asks, outlining the usual plan for treatment of a simple pneumonia. "She can go home once we do that."

"Frances is not a normal child," Sangeeta smiles even as she shakes her head. "Something else will go wrong. She always comes in with pneumonia and then ends up staying for some other reason after we get the pneumonia under control. She'll get sicker and she'll stay, and I want you to know that up front so that you know that it's not your fault."

Sangeeta is remarkably prescient in this prediction. Frances's fever breaks and then she develops diarrhea, likely from the antibiotics we are giving her for the infection. Then the frequency and length of her seizures gradually increase. Her medications are changed repeatedly but without any real response. Frances lies in bed not moving her arms or her legs, not able to even turn her head from side to side. Sometimes she smiles, but mostly she is still. Aside from the daily twitching of her tongue or one finger that signals her seizure activity, she does not stir at all. Her father, who is her mother's boyfriend and lives in a group home because of his own learning difficulties, asks for an MRI to take a picture of Frances's seizures. I explain that there is nothing we would see on an MRI that we did not see on the last CT, that her worsening seizures are not a mystery but rather quite expected, given the abnormal connections of the neurons in her brain.

Months go by. I go off service and come back to cross-cover overnight and find that no real progress has been made. Frances is still there. Although she has moved rooms several times in the intervening weeks, the story is the same. I feel a pang of sadness for her family, but it is not the same as guilt. Even if Sangeeta had not thought to tell us, I would have learned by this point that it is no one's fault that Frances does not seem to ever get better. It is just the way that she was built.

Frances is not the only child to linger in the hospital, seemingly inexplicably, for entire months at a time. She is not the only one who is broken with no hope of ever being fixed. There is a dedicated service in our hospital for children just like her. When they are not critical enough to be in the ICU, there is a special group of doctors, nurse practitioners, and social workers to care for them on the floor. These patients are among the most complicated patients in the hospital, and many of them are sick right from birth. When I rotate on CCS, the doctors have recently altered the meaning of this designation from coordinated care service to complex care service. They did not relish being treated like secretaries, called on to organize meetings among the various subspecialty physicians involved in each child's care; despite the name change, though, this is a large part of what they still inevitably must do.

The typical CCS player, as these patients were commonly called, has a seizure disorder and all too often significant developmental delay. Like Frances, he does not eat because he lacks the coordination and muscle tone to propel food from his mouth effectively into his esophagus using his tongue. He does not take a bottle because, despite being like an infant in so many other ways, he does not have the reflex needed to suck. If he is given food, it makes him choke. This aspiration of applesauce or puréed squash into his respiratory system causes recurrent pneumonias, so he is often not fed by mouth at all. Instead, he has a piece of gastric tubing that runs through his abdominal wall and empties into his stomach. He does not complain about the absence of stimulation on his taste buds because he doesn't know what he is missing, does not have the mental ability to register the loss. His brain has been damaged by lack of oxygen at the time of his birth, or it did not develop properly because when the genetic cards had been shuffled, he had been dealt a losing hand. He continues to have seizures, sometimes daily, despite the antiepileptics. He may have had a tracheostomy, a surgical opening at the base of his throat that is a secure airway, because he cannot effectively swallow even his own saliva or because during his seizures his tongue completely blocks the passage of air down into his lungs. Without these interventions patients like Frances would not survive. They would live for a while. With each passing day or month, their lungs would get weaker, would slowly be overcome by infection, and then they would peacefully pass away.

The mothers of these patients likely had experienced pregnancies like any other. They had been filled with hope and anticipation of so many things—the proms, the driver's learning permit, the first time at a sleepover with friends. But they had fallen short and been replaced by something different, something that was hopefully filled with just as much love and with small miracles and dreams that could be adjusted to fit the child that was their own.

This is the sort of child who finds his way to the CCS, which is overseen by a group of physicians who run the outpatient clinic as well as the two doctors who specialize in this population's inpatient care. It is the sort of child who, after evaluation in the ER for a common cold, is likely to be admitted simply by virtue of having too many concurrent issues to believe at first glance that he is still alive. It is also the sort of child who, in the wake of that cold, is most likely to develop a pneumonia, to have an increase in his seizures, or to contract a mysterious and indolent bacterial infection, so he appears—with more focus and intent than he has ever mustered before in his short life—to be definitively and effectively trying to die. It is this group of children who are the lepers of today, much as if in some form of internal exile they are trapped within their own faulty bodies and set apart from the world. They are at once identifiable, strapped tightly into their wheelchairs so that they do not slump forward and fall, moving only in concert with their oxygen or feeding bags or other accoutrement of sickness. On the street or in the grocery store, people stop and stare, not outright, because decorum forbids it, but covertly out of the corners of their eyes.

The physicians who care for such children after they leave the NICU are probably as close as medicine gets to making saints. To care for such a child is a burden, and it was this burden I was thinking of that first month of my internship when I wondered if it might be easier (painfully and perversely) if Connor—born far too soon and with so many complications still ahead of him—were allowed to die. But while the lives of these girls and boys are spent in doctors' offices and waiting rooms, dependent on a dozen different medications given faithfully six times a day, an endless tedium punctuated only by weeks or months spent in the hospital, they are lives their families doggedly protect. These families are the quiet heroes, the mothers and fathers endlessly riding the hospital elevator and standing with clasped hands, the medical foster parents who have taken in those children abandoned by their blood relatives and in state custody, and the single mothers trying desperately to find time to tuck in their other sons and daughters despite the overwhelming demands that become their daily routine.

Within this CCS population, the Embassy patients in particular sometimes sit for months and years at a stretch. They never go home because home is many thousands of miles away. They are largely patients from the Middle East who have been flown to this country to undergo surgeries or be trialed on medications that they could not receive otherwise. It is a foreign land that they are brought to, the stale tiled hallways of the airport and the hospital so unlike the pungent desert, that vast flat stretch of sand that has been warmed by the sun, to which they truly belong. They come to receive the very best in medical care, but because the hospital is reimbursed so generously by their governments for their inpatient stays, there is no impetus to send them elsewhere even when a transfer to a rehabilitation facility or a school for special needs would be more appropriate. Instead, they linger on the CCS inpatient service while awaiting the next procedure in a long list of stopgap measures that keep these children precariously coasting on. They sit, when lifted out of bed into a special chair, or else they lie and they listen to the radio or the television if one of these happens to be switched on, but they are all too often alone.

"The Embassy pays," Sangeeta says with great invective because the International Office is being less than helpful in processing the paperwork needed to send one of our patients home. This little boy is just over a year old and has spent all of this time in the hospital recovering from the circumstances of his birth. Aban had been the donor in a twin-to-twin transfusion, had shared a single placenta with his twin, and had much of his blood flow stolen away. Because of this he had not developed well, grew only slowly during his gestation, and then was born too small. Given this wretched start, his progress over the following year was quite remarkable. He did not die, which in itself was quite a feat. He gained weight. And though he continued to have frequent breathing difficulties that were at times more than alarming, he kept breathing nonetheless. He learned to smile. Although he did not learn to roll over or sit up or walk as his twin was doing, he did learn to kick one leg against a large plastic button in order to trigger his mother's recorded voice.

"I love you," the voice said in English.

And the stiff but reassuringly chubby leg would strike out again.

"Aban," she said as the side of his foot hit the button, but she was not there.

"This is our vacation," his parents had said when they arrived in the United States.

They had been caring for a very sick child they were not sure would live and they had neglected Aban's brother all those days and nights they had sat with him in their own NICU before he was flown to the United States. They needed a break. They needed to spend time with their other child. And so no one had asked questions when Aban was in his room alone for several days at a time. They did not ask questions when his parents came to visit only to leave one or two hours after they had arrived.

The nurses leaned over his crib and cooed. When months had passed and he had grown stronger, they put him in a car seat and brought him to the nursing station so that he would not always be alone. Then his first birthday came and his parents were still absent more often than they were not. For a while people were still silent, but they were beginning to get angry. In the whispered conversations that were conducted at his cribside, they used the word *neglect.* They understood that there was another infant to care for, but they could not bring themselves to believe that this made it all right. They knew that it was difficult, but still they wanted his parents to show they loved Aban as much as his nurses and doctors had grown to.

When I come onto the service, Sangeeta has tried four times (always unsuccessfully) to send Aban home to the hotel room the Embassy is paying for and in which his parents have been staying for the past nine months. When Sangeeta tells us that the Embassy pays, she says it angrily because she knows that it paradoxically means Aban is not getting the kind of care he actually deserves. The hospital is not the best place for a child, where he will spend long stretches at a time lying in his crib with no one to hand him toys or speak to him, to encourage him to reach for things or learn to play. But without a financial incentive to hire more staff to wade through the piles of paperwork needed to obtain permission from the Embassy to transfer him to a more appropriate facility for children with special needs (with fewer doctors and nurses but more occupational and physical therapists), it somehow is never done. He lies in his crib recovering from one illness or another until he is just well enough that Sangeeta hopes against all hope that she might be able to send him home. The hospital is also not the safest place for a child as fragile as Aban, and each time his parents had failed to visit for several days after being called to pick him up, he had fallen sick again.

As my time on CCS progresses, I realize it is not because his parents are callous and do not care for Aban that they never come to retrieve him. It is because they are frightened. They are scared of his noisy breathing and his twenty medications and the tube through which he's fed. Though they learn the medication doses and schedule and they have filled all his prescriptions, they only become more overwhelmed as the deadline for discharge approaches. When once again the day arrives, there is some excuse about a stomach bug or a cold that his twin has caught. They are trying to protect him, they say, and perhaps they really believe that this is so. But there have been too many other times Aban was meant to leave the hospital and this had happened before. Then he would pick up some virus from another patient and another month would suddenly be gone.

If he had been American, his doctors would have considered involving the Department of Children and Families. We talk about this on rounds one morning before we try to send him home again. Sangeeta is angry, but we all agree to give it one more chance. Aban's discharge is pushed back yet again. He finally goes home eight days later. He is there for forty-eight hours before his parents bring him to the emergency room. Because his situation is so complicated, he is sent up to the floor. He stays in the hospital for several days and then is sent home. Again this time it is only just a day before he comes back.

"This is just Aban," Sangeeta had told the home nurse by phone and then told the doctors who cared for him in the ER.

Still he had been admitted for his noisy breathing and his unstable heart rate and all of the other complications that make him seem such a mess.

"He is stable in his own way," Sangeeta said, meaning that although he was not normal, at least he could hold his own.

Upon this admission, Aban is placed in a double room with an infant who has respiratory syncytial virus, a particularly nasty cause of the common cold. When he inevitably picks up the virus, he is sent to the ICU and an endotracheal tube is placed down his throat because it has become too difficult for him to breathe.

"We broke him," I say to Sangeeta, because I do not believe he would have gotten this sick if his parents had kept him at home.

"Yes," she says, and this time she does not remind me that he was broken already. "I'm afraid this time we did."

The hospital is where we live. We leave our families and we go into work every morning to a job that is harrowing on the best of days and eviscerating on the worst. We do this for a time as residents because there are things we need to learn and we have promised these years to the hospital in exchange for the skills and knowledge we will need to practice with aptitude and with compassion on the other side. It is a choice. Even so, we oftentimes regret it.

Aban's parents had made a similar choice on his behalf when they decided to have him live; against all odds and at significant cost, they chose to keep their son alive. In exchange, they, too, had to live inside the hospital if they wanted to be by their son's side. But ironically, a hospital is not a healthy place. It stifles and it alienates. When Aban's parents took him home, they failed, because he was not really theirs. They had never taken ownership of him in the way that parents must with a new child, realizing at two a.m. the exact tone of voice needed to soothe or the different cries that signify hunger or discomfort or fear. Aban was special and he was fragile, but he was still their child. With every bath or feeding or diaper change that they missed, they drifted farther and farther away until—and this is not surprising—they did not know how to find their own way back. They needed to meet their son and fall in love with him all over again, this time for the boy he actually was and not the dream that he had been.

Briony, unlucky in so many ways, is blessed with a mother who is constantly at her side. She is eighteen months old when I meet her and she cannot stand. Several months earlier she had been able to pull herself upright using the bars of her crib or her mother's pale freckled hands. Then one day, instead of walking, she had fallen down, moving backward and losing this developmental milestone.

Unlike many of the other CCS children, Briony does not have cerebral palsy from an anoxic injury to her brain. But she has many other problems instead.

After countless surgeries, Briony's most pressing issue is her poor nutrition. She had been born with serious defects in her GI tract. The hole that had existed between her trachea and her esophagus was repaired in the first few days of life. Briony had an imperforate anus, a failure of her colon and rectum to meet up with the skin on the outside. In order to temporarily repair this, she had a surgery to bring part of her bowel to the surface of her abdomen, a glistening rim of moist pink mucosa where before smooth white skin had been. She was fed formula through a gastric tube and stooled through this ileostomy opening into a bag. The next surgery Briony has before her, the final reconstruction of her rectum and anus and the reconnection of intestine and colon so that she can poop from her bottom, cannot be performed until she has grown bigger. The considerable healing her body must be prepared for will not come easily with her nutrition as poor as it is.

When I meet her, Briony has lost weight, so her mother refuses to go home. Her mother has become a bookkeeper for her only daughter's health, tabulating each ounce taken in and every drop of liquid excreted out. Briony's GI tract ends at a wet pink opening in her side just above her left hip. Within the clear plastic bag that is taped to her skin over this orifice to collect Briony's watery stools, her mother places cotton balls. These cotton balls are then placed in her wet diapers and weighed every time that she is changed. Each gram is accounted for. Each decimal point is marked down in pen. It is what the nurses do for her while she is in the hospital, but it is not something we would ever ask a family to continue at home. We would, in fact, discourage this degree of vigilance, this transformation of her relationship with her daughter into one of sterile utility instead of loving caregiver, this reduction of her child into numbers recorded in marble-patterned composition notebooks, documentation of each hour of each day. Watching her pore over these volumes, it seems possible she has forgotten her daughter is not only a collection of calories in and milliliters out but also a towheaded and miniature doll who sits upright and cries at the sight of strangers, struggling to do anything as simple as crawl away.

While Briony stays in the hospital so that we can feed her, can increase the caloric density of her formula and watch to make sure that she is able to gain weight, she is transferred briefly to the ICU for monitoring following a routine and previously scheduled bronchoscopy, a procedure to look at the site of her trachea repair. All goes well and the following afternoon she is sent back to the floor. I speak briefly with the nurse practitioner in the ICU who is signing her out.

"We haven't made any changes," the female voice tells me over the phone. "She was a bit fussy because of her teething and so we gave her some Orajel and that seemed to help."

I look over her active orders in the computer and update them to include the Orajel, a pain reliever that can be rubbed directly onto aching gums. When Briony arrives on the floor, I stop by her room and congratulate her mother that the procedure has gone well. It is only a few hours later that I receive an urgent page to return to Briony's room. Briony is in her mother's arms and she is screaming. There are several nurses inside the room with her, but despite the oxygen tubing that is misting close against her face, Briony is blue. She is a color no child should ever be. Because her mother is jostling her back and forth in an effort to calm her, the oxygen probe picks up only intermittently, but when there is a clear tracing on the screen to indicate that it is working, the displayed number reads 82 instead of the high 90s where she should be.

The nurses want me to give them instructions immediately, but I do not know what to do. I do not call a Code Blue, although Briony's dusky coloring would certainly suggest a poetic symmetry if I were to go to this most extreme of measures. However, she does not appear to be dying; she is making too much noise. I order a portable chest X-ray and an albuterol neb. I listen to her screaming lungs and then I call for help. I dial the direct number for the senior resident whom I had passed only moments before at a desk just down the hall. Rebecca arrives in less than a minute and asks the nurses to get a racemic epinephrine neb. It is a medication that is given to children with upper airway narrowing like croup, an obstruction that could certainly occur from the irritation of passing a camera down her trachea during the bronchoscopy from which she has just recovered. It is not what Briony needs—if she had been having stridor, we would have heard the noise in her throat with each sharp intake of air. Nor would she have been crying with such volume. But the medicine will not hurt her at least. It is Rebecca who confirms in the first moments of her assessment that which I had not been sure: that Briony was in bigger trouble than I was expected to know how to handle.

She turns to one of the now five or six nurses milling about the room and the hall just outside: "Call the operator and tell them we have an ICU stat."

The senior ICU fellow is a short Asian man I remember from my time in the unit, although at that moment I cannot remember his name. He arrives in the room while the racemic epinephrine neb is being held in front of Briony's face. Her coloring has not improved and the oxygen saturation on the monitor has stayed essentially the same.

I feel superfluous, conspicuously useless in the hubbub that surrounds me, the pointless commotion of people essentially standing around.

"We need an ABG," the ICU fellow says.

He is asking for an arterial blood gas, a test to determine the pH and the amount of oxygen and carbon dioxide being carried in Briony's blood.

"One of the nurses is getting the kit," Rebecca tells him, because she had, in fact, thought of this before his arrival and sent someone to gather the necessary needles and syringe.

"I had just put some Orajel on her gums," Briony's mother says.

She explains that on the previous day while in the ICU, Briony had had a similar drop in her oxygen sats shortly after the numbing medication had been rubbed onto her gums. This had not been communicated to me in the brief sign-out I had received over the phone; either it had not been thought pertinent in the wake of her procedure (reason enough for her to have dropped her sats) or it had been lost in translation somewhere along the way. The Orajel is clearly an important clue, but I am still unsure what it signifies. I feel as though someone has condescended to explain the meaning of a joke, slowly and with words a kindergartener should understand, and I have still missed the punchline.

"We need to send the blood for a methemoglobin level as well as an ABG. Can you order that?" the fellow asks the nurse who is manning a portable computer station just outside the door.

I have a vague sense that I have heard this term before or have seen it written down, but any effort I make to find a connection to some sort of meaning is in vain as Briony is placed back in her crib.

"You will need to pull back on the syringe," the fellow tells me unnecessarily as he prepares the kit with which we will collect her blood, for this at least I know.

He positions the needle in the air above Briony's wrist as he feels for her radial pulse with the other hand. This butterfly needle has two plastic wings and he grasps them lightly as he advances toward the artery beneath her skin. I wait for the flash as he pulls back and then advances the point again. When I finally see this sign that he has found her artery, I pull back on the plunger to bring the blood through the tubing into the syringe.

There are at least eight other people in the room and they are whispering as the blood comes out.

"Look at the color."

"It looks like chocolate."

"Is he sure he hit the artery?"

The blood does, in fact, give the appearance of chocolate syrup instead of being a brilliant red. I try to remember this description, written somewhere in a book and likely in association with that thing called methemoglobinemia, but I still feel far from confident that I truly know what is going on.

"Let's get her downstairs," the fellow says. As quickly as this crisis had started, it is over and Briony is gone.

I excuse myself to copy over her orders onto paper, as the policy surrounding transfers assigns this responsibility to me. While I am writing, I steal a moment to look up methemoglobinemia and the long list of medications that have been known to trigger this buildup of an ineffective form of hemoglobin, of which Orajel is one. Briony had been blue because her red cells couldn't absorb oxygen and she had been crying because every muscle and tissue in her body was beginning to burn. I bring her orders down to the unit and find that she has been given methylene blue, the antidote I just read of and finally remember learning about when patients were still abstract entities and not little girls in lavender overalls. In the ICU she has stopped crying. The toxicology fellow is sitting at the desk just outside the bay into which Briony's crib has been moved. She gives me a few articles and case reports on methemoglobinemia. I look through them as I walk back to the pile of paperwork I had left behind when Briony first had turned blue.

The following day, Kate, one of our chief residents, stops me as I am passing by the office that she shares with the other two chiefs who work at Children's.

"I heard about your methemoglobinemia baby," she tells me. I am not surprised. Rare conditions and the frightening events they inspire are always discussed afterward. "I wanted to let you know that you did a great job."

I shake my head and exhale part of a reluctant laugh.

"All I did was call for help," I tell her in protest. "I've never dialed so fast before in my life."

"You're not expected to always know what to do," Kate replies earnestly. "You're expected to know when you're in over your head and then to get the right people there to help you as quickly as you can. You did that. You did exactly your job."

I appreciate Kate's words, but they are little consolation in light of this latest reminder that I still have so much to learn. There are still gaps, and they are significant, between expectation and execution. There had been a look of condemnation on the face of the first nurse I had met eyes with as I had walked into Briony's room. She had seemed to blame me, even in those first two or three seconds, for not already knowing what she had taken ten minutes to figure out: that Briony was in real trouble. It is likely that this nurse, for all the years of experience that she had and I didn't, was simply scared because she was just as ignorant of the key to the puzzle as I had been. Still I carried that look with me and it rankled.

It is only after another whole year has passed that I am finally able to put to good use the fear that Briony's azure color had inspired, writing an educational parody of the Britney Spears song *Toxic* for our spring talent show that explained both the symptoms of her Orajel exposure and the treatment that enabled her to get well. By the time the audio track is recorded and the resulting music video is carefully edited by Daryl, Briony is again able to stand. She has had a baby brother who is perfect and healthy and to whom she chats a mile a minute from the confines of her hospital crib. Her mother, with the addition of the new baby to their family, has had to let go of her composition notebooks. Although she still meticulously cares for Briony's G-tube site and the skin around her ostomy, she looks happier and more relaxed than I have ever seen her before.

I tell her how to find the video on YouTube and she laughs, telling me, "You've made my daughter famous."

And I respond, "She deserves to be."

*   *   *

Briony is one of the patients who makes the CCS service so rewarding, because of these hard-won victories, because of the moments when things go right. But toward the end of my month with Sangeeta and Venee, we are transferred a patient who reminds me again why I would never be able to find the strength to do this job every day. Muffinball is called by his last name in part because his first is so difficult to pronounce and also because, with the omission of the hyphen during his registration, an already incongruous surname had its absurdity amplified. He is an ex-twenty-four-week preemie who has had significant bleeding in his brain. When I first cared for him with Leisha in the ICU, he had been given a tracheostomy to breathe through and was on a ventilator for additional support. In the several intervening months between my rotation in the unit and my responsibilities on CCS, Muffinball gets worse at times and then gets better, but generally improves from a respiratory standpoint until he is breathing on his own through his trach collar with no help from a machine.

He reminds me in many ways of Connor, because Muffinball is the sort of baby I feared Connor would become. He does not give any indication that he recognizes his mother or knows when he is being held. He may even be blind. His muscles are so stiff as a result of the damage to his brain that his arms and legs are always straight. Unlike Frances, whose muscle tone is diminished to the point that she does not really move, Muffinball moves constantly but without direction or intent. He flings his tiny arms upward or sideways. On one occasion he flipped his body over, so his trach, then connected to a breathing machine, was pulled right out. There had been a brief time when his heart stopped beating before he was brought back to life.

He will never be a normal child, but it is possible, while he is still so small, to forget this and to mistake his strange dystonic dance for purpose of a kind. Muffinball's mother, Kay, does not know her son when she first starts asking questions about finally bringing him home. Like Aban, he has recently turned a year old. With the winter holidays approaching, Kay has hopes that he will be discharged in time for Christmas. I explain, as I have done before, that we need to consider a permanent feeding tube, since he is still being given formula through a thin tube run into his nose and down the back of his throat into his stomach. She could in theory be taught how to replace such a tube should it be pulled out, but eventually it will erode into his facial bones. Also, the airway congestion caused by the tube in his nose makes his already delicate respiratory status even more precarious, meaning that he is more likely to fall gravely ill the first time that he catches a cold as he is certain (in these winter months) to eventually do.

Kay has heard this before and she has said no. She will not put him through another surgery. She does not want to cause him pain. There are parents who listen to all of the options, weigh the risks, look at the kind of life their child is living, and decide that it is kinder to let the child go. It is possible that this is what Kay is doing, although I doubt it, and that she is being difficult because she does not know how to tell us what she really feels. It is a trap we set for parents without meaning to, telling them what the next step is without at the same time reminding them that the next step does not have to come. We believe we are doing them a kindness, and that in the face of caring for such a complicated daughter or son, optimism is the least of all the things that they deserve. The danger then is that parents will be ashamed to disappoint, to admit when they are beginning to give up hope. On the other side of this same coin, however, is the pain that is inflicted by physicians who by their words imply to a mother or father that their child does not deserve to live. It is a thin edge that we have to aim for and one that I had negotiated badly that first month while taking care of Connor, trying to make Missy and Charles aware just how sick he was, believing it was my responsibility to make this clear to them in case they wanted something less than everything, wanted to erase the line and draw it somewhere else instead.

"We have to push because that's our job," I tell another family, a mother and a grandmother of a little boy who has a social smile, a skill that is learned at three months of age, but whose development never progressed beyond that. "But you know Kyle better than we do and so that means that it is absolutely your place to push right back. We know that Kyle will not live for as long as other people and we are trying to give him the best life that he can have. If there is ever a surgery or other procedure that we suggest but you don't think is right for him, then you need to tell us. You need to say when it's too much, when it's time to just say no."

For once I had read the silent cues correctly and they had thanked me, had looked almost relieved at this affirmation of what they had suspected but had been unable to discuss—that there is a cost to everything we do.

Kay is right to be protective of her son, because placing a permanent feeding tube in Muffinball's abdomen means a major surgery. The simpler G-tubes that many of the other CCS patients get, where an endoscope is threaded down the esophagus to the stomach wall and then the tube is popped through to the other side, is not a procedure for which Muffinball is a candidate. Again, like Connor, as one of the many complications of his early birth he had lost large segments of bowel, parts of his gut that had died from lack of blood flow and that had had to be cut out. The resulting scarring inside his abdomen means that he needs an open surgery to place the tube and that the recovery afterward will involve significantly more pain.

"I don't think he needs the tube," Kay tells me. "The NG tube is working fine for now."

She is holding Muffinball sideways in her lap so that his arching back is draped across one arm instead of pushing against her chest. She cannot sit him straight because he will not stay bent at the hips but rather thrusts his pelvis forward as if he is trying to get down.

I remind her that the nasogastric tube is only a temporizing measure and that it has already been in for far too long.

"Why don't you feed him then?" she says in a voice that has a hint of accusation.

"Through his mouth?" I ask, unsure that I have understood.

Muffinball's tongue pushes forward and licks his lips and then is pulled back again. This movement, not at all voluntary, repeats every few seconds. Months ago, he had a workup for possible epilepsy, which showed brain activity that was incredibly abnormal but that was not a seizure we could treat. He moves his tongue just as he moves his arms and legs, because the part of his brain that governs gross motor skills is damaged and is constantly going off.

When I speak with Sangeeta, we decide that it is worth the risk to feed him. He may aspirate. He may have respiratory compromise. But while he is in the hospital, he is relatively safe, and it makes good sense to see what he will do. When a bottle is put in his mouth, he sucks, but quickly after this, his tongue pushes the nipple away. It is the same with a spoon carrying puréed vegetables and fruits. He takes in some calories by mouth, but it is only a tiny fraction of what he needs to grow. The rest we continue to run through his NG tube until eventually Kay is satisfied that the experiment, at least for the time, has failed.

"I want to get him home," she says when she finally agrees to meet with the surgeons to talk about the feeding tube. "I know that he needs to grow right now and that it's what we need to do."

What she means is that she understands that he cannot eat enough by mouth right now. However, she still maintains he someday will.

"When will the surgeons come?"

I tell her.

"And the ophthalmologists? He still hasn't had his full exam."

This had been an ongoing struggle since Muffinball and I were in the unit together, and it still has not been resolved. It is not for lack of trying on either our part or the ophthalmologists'. On one occasion they had come to do their exam and had snidely told us to call them to come back when he wasn't seizing. In addition to the tongue thrusting, Muffinball's eyeballs roll back in his head. They are always moving, although his lids are down. When you pull the eyelid open, his gaze swivels around to right or left.

"He must be blind," Venee had commented once, "or else he would be throwing up."

"We'll certainly keep trying to arrange it," I tell Kay in response to her questioning. "You remember they've tried to do the exam several times but haven't been able to."

"I need to know if he can see," she explains. "I'm going to be moving apartments before he comes home. Section 8 is helping me get another room. I'm probably going to be looking at places later this month and I don't want to have to move again. I need to know what to look for if a blind child will be living there."

As she speaks, I have the slow but sickening realization of what she is trying to say.

"Why does it matter?" I ask just to be sure.

"There can't be funny corners or stairs from one room to the next. It wouldn't be safe."

It is likely that when he was in the NICU his doctors did not expect him to live. It is possible they never said anything. Remembering how difficult it was to broach the subject with Missy and Charles, I cannot blame them if they had remained silent. Or it is possible that they mustered the courage to speak, as I had so clumsily tried to do, but Kay simply didn't hear. To ignore what should have been so obvious is all too easy, with both parent and doctors garnering the same focus and optimism with which we daily check items off a to-do list, but this positive motion has now unforgivably let Kay and her child down. We have kept Muffinball alive against the odds, yet in the midst of all of the tubes and surgeries and procedures, we never told the truth.

"I don't think he'll ever walk," I tell her as gently but as firmly as I can.

"Why do you say that?" her face making it obvious that this is not a possibility she has considered.

"He's a year old now and he doesn't roll over. He doesn't sit. He doesn't reach for things even if you brush them up against him to let him know that they are there. He doesn't have control over the way his arms and legs are moving. He's absolutely made incredible progress and is a very strong little boy, but there are things that other children learn that he will never do."

When we meet later in the week with all of the teams involved in Muffinball's care, Kay asks the neurologist who has looked over his old MRIs, "Do you think it's right, what people are saying, that he may never walk?"

The neurologist, a small elderly man who exudes empathy as if from his pores, uses a soft and placid tone, but he says the words *brain damage* in no uncertain terms.

"I understand that he may not do everything that normal babies do, but he'll do the best he can. I'm going to help him at least do that," Kay tells us. I realize that with this statement she has finally started to own and love her son for who he really is.

When I pass Sangeeta in the hall a few weeks later, she tells me, "Your boyfriend finally left," meaning Muffinball.

I had already noticed that his name had been taken down from his room and had been replaced. It had not been in time for Christmas or in time for the start of the New Year, but even so, he was gone. Against incredible odds his mother had taken him home. He will require care around the clock to keep him growing. It will be a job that Kay will shoulder for the duration of his life because he will never really grow any older than he is now.

There are some patients on the service who are almost the same age as I am. The parents keeping watch over their hospital beds could be my own. In place of high school and college and medical school graduations, there have been hospital admissions and discharges, CTs, and orthopedic surgeries. In place of choir concerts, there have been diaper changes. In place of trips to the Galápagos or Europe to foot the bill for, there have been new wheelchairs or a special-order brace. There are times that I cry for these families, in secret, as I am sure that they would resent the pity. Still on rounds the tears well quickly and have to be blinked away.

More than a year later, I will pass a room with Aban's name outside the door and inside it will be as empty of family members as it ever was, and I will worry again about what his future will hold. Muffinball, though sicker in so many ways and unable to laugh or even meet his mother's gaze, I do not worry about at all. I know that it is possible that he will live into his twenties or even beyond, that there might be decades of diaper changes and tube feedings and around-the-clock care ahead. And while I know that it will certainly be difficult, I feel strangely confident that Kay will still have the strength throughout it all to remain at his side.

Surfacing

When enough time has gone past, there are places that I come back to again. I enter an elevator or step through a doorway, not with the sense of ease that should follow from habit, but as a swimmer might—with both trepidation and excitement—leave behind the sandy shallows to explore deeper water. I move through each scene with a sense of disorientation and blurred edges as if it has already happened, as if it already belongs to memory and is locked in the past. In the present there should be the sharp definition of a hot sun and a vast cloudless sky, the warmth holding in place the long brown bodies stretched on the scorching sand just out of reach of gentle saltwater waves. But instead of coral or shells or the darting bodies of brightly colored fish, the objects I meet again are cardiovascular monitors and ventilator machines, sat probes and IV pumps. Though they are just as I remember them, they are still somehow unreal, even though they feel solid, cool to the touch. These things are smaller, as if observed from a distance, and as I walk into the NICU to take on my new role, carrying the Delivery Room pager, I pause at the spot where Connor's tiny form once had been.

It has been almost a year since I last looked through his records, a year and a half since that brief four-week stretch when he had felt so entirely mine. When I had last looked in his chart, it was just after Connor's first birthday, and the notes there outlined the progress he had made in that first year of his life. The next time I am sitting in front of a computer and find myself thinking of him, I realize I have forgotten his father's last name, the name he had taken upon his release from the hospital after a 131-day stay. Without this, I cannot open his electronic chart, cannot check one more time that he is, in fact, alive. Lingering for a moment in the spot I had so often stood during those first weeks of my internship, I feel again like a wave of nostalgia the certainty that Connor would die. It was a feeling that I had not questioned, that I had nurtured even, believing as I did that such harsh acceptance was necessary and meant I was ready for all that the three years of residency would bring. But Connor had not died during that month when he was in my care and he did not die in the following weeks and months. He was not well. We had not been untruthful when we warned his parents of the things they should expect. Missy and Charles, though they had seemed not to listen to so many of the things that we said, had cared for this child with his tubes and his surgeries that I had so often worried they would not want.

Where Connor had been, there is now an infant on CPAP (continuous positive airway pressure), the two prongs in her nose delivering pressurized air. Connor would have gone through this transition after he was weaned from his ventilator but not yet ready to breathe reliably just on room air. He would have been several months old by that time. In contrast, the infant I am now watching was born only two days before. She is near-term or even just beyond it. If it is only her breathing that is causing her problems, she will quickly be released to go home. These are the infants who are loved without the cold certainty of heartbreak, the ones who will surely recover from the slight immaturity of their lungs. This hospitalization is a brief blip of unsteadiness in the normal childhood that they have ahead. They are children who would struggle had they been born in other countries, who would have had to fight for life and who might have lost. They are the ones who exist without blurred edges, the ones I know we should save. But there are others in the room, I see now as I survey more closely, who are like Connor, who are little more than paper-thin purple skin stretched over organs that are not yet fully formed. Their kidneys dump electrolytes and their livers cannot process the bilirubin released during the destruction of their red blood cells, turning the whites of their eyes a sickly yellow, prompting the banks of blue-tinged lights directed at their skin. In one corner an infant I estimate to be about 3 pounds moons the passersby, his thin legs folded beneath his abdomen to raise his bare bottom in the air, keeping it as dry as possible to allow his diaper rash to heal.

After a moment, I walk down the hall and leave this room behind. Beyond this bay that holds the sickest children is the room in which those who are nearing discharge are moved before they can go home. It is the equivalent of babysitting and I am there only to occasionally look in on the nurses who know how to do this job much better than I ever will. It is the nurses who sit chatting at the center of this sunny space that has windows on two sides, rocking slowly back and forth the infants tucked beneath their arms. They change diapers and give bottles to those who are just learning to suck. When one of these small charges, each nearing his or her due date, lets out a breath and forgets to take another, it is the nurses who are there to firmly rub the child's back and trigger the next sharp intake of air. I am not needed here, except on the rare occasion when things go unexpectedly wrong. I am called only once in the time that I am on this rotation to the bedside of a baby boy whose heart is pumping much too quickly. I have to press ice onto his face and push a medication into his vein to slow it down.

My primary responsibilities are the deliveries that take place on the floor below, that require I be ready at any moment to storm down the stairs through the operating or delivery room doors. It is the same staircase I had rushed down more than eighteen months earlier, when Kate, Neil, and Laura had raced just steps ahead. The joke on that day had been that we might be required to take the instruments that Alli had handed to us and slip them past the white fish mouth of a struggling infant's vocal cords. I am not sure when it was meant to have happened, this transition from mockery to real expectation, but I know that it had come. When I reach the end of the hall, it is with a practiced motion that I slip the first-call pager over the bunched-up cloth at the drawstring waist of my fresh blue scrubs and flip a red neonatal stethoscope to hang around my neck.

In the delivery room there is a woman pushing as her husband whispers in her ear. I knock before I enter, then move as quietly as possible toward the warmer and wave my hand beneath the lights to check that they are on. I flip open the laryngoscope to make sure the bulb is working and close the blade again, lifting the thin mattress just enough to slide the metal instrument underneath. Beside it, I slip the ET tube I have just opened, still within its plastic wrapper, the guide wire I have inserted bent over the top. I quickly slide my eyes over the suction bulb lying on the sterile blankets, the suction controls mounted on the wall. It takes perhaps a minute and then I stand motionless, leaning against the wall. I wait, moving only occasionally and as inconspicuously as I can to look between the woman's legs. I am there because a gush of meconium-stained fluid had soaked through the bedsheets when her water finally broke. When I look, I see an oval of dark brown hair matted with thick yellow mucus and clotted flecks of blood.

The first time I had stood before this process, it had taken hours from the time the hair had first become visible until the head finally emerged, larger than I had ever imagined it would be. Now I know that it is unpredictable, how quickly a labor will progress, and I have been called in for only the final moments when the obstetrician will slip her hands around the infant's neck to deliver first one shoulder and then the next. When she does this, the child immediately screams and I pull the laryngoscope, no longer needed, from its hiding place and drop it into the pocket of my scrub shirt. The instrument technically does not belong to this department but to the NICU, and I will need to bring it upstairs to be sterilized. The OB holds the infant suspended in her hand, draped over her gloved palm, while the umbilical cord is cut. Then she places the still shrieking newborn onto a towel spread over his mother's chest. The nurses rub the child clean as I watch from my position on the wall. The infant's father wipes a hand across his eyes and plants a tender kiss on the forehead of his new son. As soon as I am satisfied that the infant is breathing comfortably, I duck out as quietly, I hope, as I had first come in.

On the tenth floor a woman has been admitted who has just entered her thirty-second week. It is my job to meet with this couple and explain the things they have in store. She is not in active labor yet and has not been moved to the floor the delivery rooms are on, but she has had several small contractions and is receiving IV hydration to see if they can be stopped. Before I go to see her, I flip though the binder that contains an overview of everything that I should say.

The expectant mother is petite and slender, so the belly—despite the month it should have ahead to grow bigger still—dominates her tiny frame, floating above her and partially blocking her face when I stand at the foot of the hospital bed. Her husband presses his thumb onto the bed railing and a motor grinds into motion and raises her head until she can look me in the eye. I introduce myself and explain that it is our policy to always meet with parents if there is a possibility that they will deliver prematurely.

"I know there's still a good chance that they'll send you home and you won't deliver your baby until it is time, but if you do end up delivering today I want to go over the sort of things you can expect."

Without warning she is crying and her husband is slipping a tissue into her hand. I know this look and I have seen it before. It is not the hormones or the stress or the million other things about this woman's day that are so far from what she hoped they would be. It is *me*, standing before her, that brings the tears so quickly to her eyes. I have a giraffe embroidered on my fleece jacket and a stethoscope designed to rest on a chest that is only the width of my left hand. I know that just my being in her room makes this real for her in a way that nothing else up until this moment could have done. I am a doctor and she has seen many of these in the preceding months, but I am not here for her. I am what comes after the labor and the delivery. I am the first pediatrician whom she has met.

I wait for her to blow noisily into the rough tissue and to wipe the balled wad of paper across her nose.

"What I need to say first and most importantly is that babies delivered at thirty-two weeks usually do very well. If you don't remember anything else that I tell you, I want you to remember that. Thirty-two weeks is early—you already know that—but by and large, most of the babies born at this age end up healthy and beautiful babies."

She sniffles again into a second tissue and attempts a smile.

"Thank you," she says.

"You don't need to thank me," I tell her. "You've done a wonderful job getting this far. I should also tell you right from the start that if the infant is born today, or born anytime up until thirty-five weeks gestation, that he or she will have to come to the neonatal intensive care unit or the NICU no matter how great he or she is doing. That way we know that he or she is in a place with the best nurses and plenty of pediatricians right there making sure that everything continues to look good."

I pause, then ask, "Do you know if you're having a boy or a girl?"

The woman's husband squeezes her hand and answers, "We're having a little girl."

"That's wonderful," I tell them, "although little boys are lovely, too, but to be honest, girls who are born early tend to do a little bit better with their breathing early on, and obviously the way your baby is breathing is going to be one of the first things we worry about. I'm going to explain a whole bunch of things, so please interrupt me if you have any questions or if there's something that I haven't made very clear."

I talk for almost twenty minutes about CPAP and ventilators and the way premature lungs need support until they are developed enough to work. I explain how, even if their daughter does need to be intubated, they will still get to hold her in their arms. The couple nods occasionally, but they do not speak. What I do not say but I know they understand is that whatever happens, should she be delivered this early, we will be taking her away, that all of the things I am outlining are things we may have to do while they are not there to see. I tell them how babies born early are often given antibiotics because of the chance that an infection in the placenta triggered the premature labor. I explain how sometimes premature infants need to have a picture taken of their heart using an ultrasound in just the same way that ultrasounds had been done to watch the progress of the fetus as it was getting bigger each day inside.

Finally, I admit that premature infants are incredibly bad at feeding, at sucking down enough calories to keep them gaining a little bit of weight each and every day. It is the feeding that is likely to keep infants in the hospital even after their breathing has improved. The baby will suck slowly, choke, turn red, and may even need a temporary feeding tube threaded down from her nose. Watching this will be very frustrating, once she has grown plumper and looks like the sort of girl Anne Geddes would place in a flowerpot or give gossamer wings, because by this time she will have gotten so close to going home that they will be able to taste it, will be able to smell her skin long after they have left the hospital. I write up my consult note, listing the topics we have covered, and leave it for the attending to sign once she has met the couple herself. I hear later that they were only kept overnight and then sent home with careful instructions to return immediately if the contractions recur.

It is in this way that my days are assembled, with long relaxed conversations meant to impart calm punctuated by the sort of activity that cannot be delayed for any but the most abbreviated of explanations. In the OR a mother is delivering by cesarean section an infant that is just twenty-four weeks along and I think once more of Connor, of how small he would have been on that day when he was born. But this infant is even smaller, and has been suffering from inadequate nutrition because it was all that its imperfectly functioning placenta could provide. Standing just outside the OR door, we can see the small dome of a belly that has been pregnant for just six months.

"If he doesn't cry, that's it—it's over—and I'm not intubating."

The attending absently passes one hand over her own belly, in which she is carrying a fetus only a few weeks younger than the one we are about to see. The unborn baby in the OR is just at that line of viability—a line that has been arbitrarily set and then pushed back further and further. His mother has been given steroids by her obstetricians to help develop his lungs, but he is still small, even for his twenty-four weeks, and giving this medication is not something the neonatologists would have recommended had they been asked. They know that he has just not grown big enough.

I leave the OR once when my pager goes off and run to the other side of the floor to a delivery at which, it turns out, I am not really needed. The attending's back is to me when I reenter the OR and her right arm lifts as she pulls straight up to remove the wire from the ET tube she has just inserted into the newborn's throat.

"He cried?" I ask.

She shrugs and says, "He squeaked," and she looks defeated.

His skin is bronzed, not from the sun, but from the blood vessels that show through. Each rib is visible as the Neopuff ventilator delivers measured minute breaths. His heart is beating rapidly. I can see each contraction of the muscle as it pushes up against the wafer-thin chest wall. There is nothing more to be done. Upstairs he will need lines inserted into the central artery and vein that are accessible in the remaining jelly of his umbilical cord, but for now he is loaded into an isolette and rolled with the ventilator to where his mother (her abdomen still open and being repaired) can reach an arm into the opening to rest over the soft curve of his head.

"He's so small," she says in disbelief. "I didn't think he could be so small."

She is visibly disturbed by the sight of him and she turns away.

"I want his father to see him before he dies," she says, and we roll the infant toward the door.

Now that he is intubated, there is no question of taking the tube out without meetings and paperwork and the family standing by. His father is at least hours away by car, but still there is no telling if the infant will last that long. His blood pressure could drop at any moment, from an infection if there is one or simply from being born too soon. As we prepare to leave the room, another attending neonatologist and a fellow run past our room. We secure the breathing tube with another piece of tape and roll the newborn into the hall. I look left toward the door that has just swung shut behind the group that had been rushing by.

"Go," my attending tells me. "We'll get this one upstairs."

I grab a fresh pair of gloves as I walk from one OR into the next, a mask covering half my face.

"I'm the junior resident," I say by way of introduction when I approach the commotion at the open warmer in the corner. "Is there anything I can do?"

"You can take over the chest compressions," I am told. This new attending instructs the fellow to move her hands away and concentrate on the infant's airway instead.

On the warmer the infant is limp with gray skin but appears to be full term. I wrap my hands around the infant's chest and press my thumbs against the sternum to compress the heart beneath.

"Count out loud," the attending tells me. I count each time I press down, interrupting the count to insert the word *breathe* and then starting again.

The fellow, who is at the infant's head and is squeezing air into her lungs, is not paying attention to the count I am reciting. Instead, she is looking over her left shoulder at the nurse, who had been the only one present when the baby had come out.

"There was no history?" she is asking this other woman. "No decelerations in the heart rate?"

The eyes above the pale blue mask are frightened, but the nurse keeps her voice even and calm, knowing that behind the sterile sheet not feet away from us sits the infant's father as he holds tight to his wife's hand.

"We lost the tracing just for a few minutes before the infant emerged. Before that, it had been fine. The section was for failure to progress and she had been in labor for just over twelve hours."

The respiratory therapist takes over the bag and mask while the fellow prepares the ET tube. Then the fellow resumes her place at the infant's head and inserts the blade into the mouth.

"I need some pressure," she says.

The respiratory therapist pushes two fingers into the soft fat of the newborn girl's exposed throat to move the vocal cords into view.

"I've got it," the fellow says and leaves her finger pressed up against the hard palate of the infant's mouth to keep the tube in place.

The respiratory therapist, who I see only as a pair of large, smooth, disconnected hands and wrists, connects the anesthesia bag with its flow of oxygen to the breathing tube that has just been put in. He hands it to the fellow to squeeze while he tapes the tube quickly in place.

"Let's give a dose of epinephrine through the tube while I set up to put in a line."

"Hold compressions," the fellow tells me.

I stop the rhythmic squeezing and gently close two fingers around the base of the umbilical stump. The pulsation of blood, which should be bounding, continues to merely plod along.

"Still less than 60," I report. "I'm starting compressions again."

I count out loud and this time the fellow breathes with me. The infant, despite the way we are attacking her, still lies flaccid and does not move. I notice that her color has improved, at least, as the first dose of epinephrine is given through the breathing tube. Only inches below where my hands are resting, the attending is trying to clean the umbilical stump so that she can thread an emergency line into the vein. My left arm is extended over the infant's chest to squeeze on the right side, mirroring the hold I have on her left rib cage, and I am in the attending's way. I try to contort so that my elbow is moved forward toward the infant's head to give the attending more room to work.

"Don't change what you are doing," she says sharply, and I resume my earlier position with my left elbow bumping her shoulder as the line goes in.

She pulls back on the plunger attached to the end of the narrow thread and a flash of red mixes with the saline in the syringe. Then she pushes a few milliliters of the salt water in to be sure the line can flush.

"Get ready to give a dose of epinephrine through the line," she says.

From over the wall of shoulders, a hand is thrust with another syringe in its fist. I hear a voice repeat the dose of epinephrine that she is handing over, correctly calculated for the estimated weight of the child.

"I'm pushing the epi," the attending says. "Continue CPR."

During this span of several minutes the infant has no fewer than four sets of hands upon her at any one time. The fellow continues to deliver breaths while I compress the chest. The attending finishes securing the line and the respiratory therapist listens as each breath goes in. The next time I hold compressions, the heart rate is above 100 and my job is done. Moments later, the infant coughs and begins moving her arms.

"She's fighting it," the fellow says as she bags another breath into the now squirming infant. "What do you want to do?"

The attending considers this: "I still think we don't have a good explanation for what went wrong. It's probably safer to leave the tube in for now."

As she says this, the infant coughs again and the fellow leans further forward.

"I think it might have just come out."

The attending moves slightly from where she stands at the infant's right side and has to slide just six inches to the left to bring herself level with the newborn's fuzz-covered head.

"You think, or you know?" the attending asks, demanding a decision.

"It's out," the fellow confirms.

"Then pull it."

The respiratory therapist peels off the soft anchor of tape adhering to the side of the mouth and the fellow pulls the dislodged tube out of the throat.

The infant cries. After a few minutes of watching the girl, the attending lifts her shoulders once to signal her confusion.

"Pull the line, too, I guess. We'll still bring her upstairs."

The drapes and tubes and syringes are cleared away before the newborn's father, with much hesitation, comes to stand by her head. He rests one index finger in her now pink palm and she curls all five fingers and holds on. It is as if the interminable passage of minutes through which we had just traveled did not exist for her and she is born into this moment when she takes her father's hand.

By the time I come into the hospital the next day, the twenty-four weeker has already died. His father had lifted his small body into his own two cupped hands and signed the papers that said nothing more was to be done. They did not pull the tube and continued to give him tiny puffs of air, but even so, it was not many hours before his heart began to weary and eventually it came to rest. No one stood over him and did futile chest compressions upon a surface that was not even as wide as my own hand. They simply said goodbye and meant it; then he was let go. This is what I had imagined for Connor when I first had met him all those many months before. I had wished for him such an exit absent of pain, but it was not what had come to pass. Instead, Connor had grown. He had teetered on that thin edge between life and that thing that comes when it has ended, held tight and suspended there only in the culmination of all the technology and ingenuity that medicine had to give.

I find Margaret at the end of my first week back in the NICU, the woman who, for all the months he had been with them, was Connor's primary nurse. She is a short woman, her cheeks tanned by a recent cruise vacation, her face framed by a silver bob. She does not remember me, although she graciously pretends to, and she sighs as she thinks back on how difficult it all had been. The air escapes from between her teeth in a prolonged and even hiss. She pats a firm hand on the back of the infant she has finished feeding.

"I thought what they went through with Connor was enough. It would be enough for anyone, any couple. It's a stress that too many of them can't find reason enough to make it through. I just didn't believe when Missy got pregnant again."

My eyes are wide as Margaret reminisces. Another pregnancy is not a situation I can imagine could have ended well. Missy had at least one early miscarriage, and then, just before Connor, had carried a fetus just past twenty weeks. It happens this way sometimes. Not everyone is made to easily carry children, and there are wombs that, when stretched, open and let the life they have inside them slip away too soon. For Missy, with this sort of history, I could hardly imagine going through it again.

"What happened?" I ask with dread, but also, I have to admit, with a sick sort of anticipation.

"We were full when she delivered, so she couldn't have her here, which was hard on Missy and Charles, too. But she carried her to thirty-two weeks, bless her, and she did great as far as I know. She brought her over for a visit not long after she went home."

There is nothing more to say because I cannot say out loud how very wrong I had been. I do not need to ask for absolution despite the fact that this is how I sometimes feel. I had done my job. I had wanted what was best for Connor. I had just been wrong about what that was. So, instead, I thank Margaret for her company. I leave her with an infant draped over one shoulder and a burp cloth across the other. The chair she sits in creaks in rhythm as she rocks to and fro. It is like standing before some sage or zephyr at the narrow entrance to a fire-lit cave. There is that same promise of revelation and completion. I feel the air shifting softly around me as I wait for things to begin to become clear.

It is around this time that my grandmother dies. It had already been years since she was last well, the layering on of time and sickness, a failing body sustained only by pills and operations. Still, when it happens, it is somehow a surprise. She dies alone in a hospital bed with no one holding tight to her bony hand. There had been vigils, pilgrimages to Fort Lauderdale to the mobile home park, but they had repeatedly been premature. Now, after all of the fuss that had gone before it, the moment had been missed. My mother flies down to see to the particulars, the death certificate, the cremation. My father goes with her. It is not the sort of thing that he is good at. The paperwork, the waiting, will all try his patience. He will find it disagreeable, but I realize that it is something that must be endured. It is what family does for each other.

We wait until summer for the funeral and then drive out of the city. My grandmother's younger sister, ninety herself, has flown up from Florida for the service. It is mostly family, my aunts and uncles and cousins, but there are some aging friends of my grandmother's as well. They toddle unsteadily or else are pushed in wheelchairs up to the grassy grave. The brass plaque with my grandmother's name on it is already set into the ground. The left half also bears my grandfather's name and his years of birth and death. Arranged to either side are the plaques honoring my great grandfather and one with the name of my grandmother's youngest brother, Pete. He had been the baby of the family and an airman in the Second World War, a gunner. While he was beneath the plane, it had caught some flak but was not too badly hit. Even so, his oxygen hose was cut and he died of suffocation, without a single mark on him. His sister would outlive him by more than seventy years.

We stand in a clump at the grave marker in the late morning. My brother's wife, Marnie, reads a short passage about friendship or love or the impermanence or the permanence of something. When she returns to her place at my brother's side, I notice that Daryl is crying. He had never met my grandmother. We had meant to travel down to Florida, but we never seemed to find the time. Still he is crying openly and he does not wipe the tears away. There is his own mother he could be thinking of, or his father, both of whom are aging and neither of whom are entirely well. It may be years before he and his brother are forced to make the sort of decisions my mother has just had to make. But it will come, eventually, and when it does, there will be nothing more than a brief gathering of mourners and all of the things he never got a chance to say.

Or it is possible that it is just the sadness of it all, a sadness that is not particular to any one place or person but that is overwhelming nonetheless. We all want to hold on to what is in front of us. Missy and Charles felt it, their faces pressed against the clear walls of the isolette, their breath fogging the plastic that was in between. I had wondered what they could be thinking, why they insisted on smiling when they reached in to take Connor's purple hand. I thought it was because they were not listening, did not hear the warnings we had to give: he may not talk, he may not swallow, he may spend his life in and out of the hospital and being shuttled around in a custom-made wheelchair. But there was no way of asking. If when we spoke their faces hardened, became enough like stone that they seemed impermeable to any sort of truth aside from the one they had chosen, then there was nothing we could do. I thought that loving Connor had to mean loving all of him, acknowledging the difficulties that were to come. And someday it would come to mean this for Missy and Charles, I realized only slowly, but it was not something they could absorb right away. Back then, when he hovered so precariously between life and the thing that comes after, it was simply enough for them that Connor was still there.

More than two years after first meeting Connor, I come across the website Missy had been keeping. I find it after much searching on a quiet holiday weekend, when my pager is silent for most of my twenty-four-hour shift. There are pictures of Connor at his second birthday, smiling, thick glasses distorting his brown eyes. He is not perfect, but they are happy in these snapshots, Missy and Charles and their first child. I read about his G-tube and how he does not use it any longer, is instead eating by mouth, and is about to have it taken out. The hole in his stomach will close quickly and the skin will heal over time, leaving only a scar on a belly ridden deep with such marks but growing stronger just the same. It is impossible, I think, as I scroll down the long entries, that this is the same child I had touched only cautiously, the one who had bled so badly into his skull, whose nose and fingers had turned black. I had expected him to adopt the lifeless stares of so many of the patients who are cared for by our hospital's complex care service. With all the damage it seemed had been done, I did not believe that his eyes would ever be able to focus, that he would be able to recognize his parents at all. I remember now how that first NICU attending with whom I had worked had summed up this powerlessness, this absolute inability to ever truly achieve prescience: "Sometimes you just can't tell."

On the right side of the web page there is a vertical banner with a link to Missy's other blogs. I click the one at the top, labeled with the names of her little girl.

"We're having another baby!" Missy writes in the first entry. "We just went to the doctor today. I know how hard it was for us to keep you all updated after Connor was born so I thought I'd start this new blog now." Then, "Week 7: We just had our first ultrasound and heard the heartbeat! We're going out to dinner at Ninety-nine with Connor to celebrate so I don't have time to write more now."

"Week 12: No more doctors offices for me this week. Connor had two appointments yesterday and it was just about all that I could take. Sometimes I wonder how we can be thinking about starting all over again."

It is there, after all, the small sense of doubt that I had so often searched for and had not found. Perhaps it had been there the whole time, hidden away, covered over in its hard shell casing like a nut lodged in the bottom of her throat. I had thought she was not listening, but instead she was saving them for later, this collection of possibilities, doubts, and fears. Maybe she had taken them out when she was alone with Connor in those first few months that he was home, when he was crying for his feeding to be hung. It would have been a frightening transition for Missy, the responsibility of such a small sick creature after the months in the NICU having nothing really to do. Certainly she must have questioned during those months of her pregnancy whether this was something she could live through again. She must have doubted, but like so many of the other parents I had watched in their vigils, she daily summoned the strength it took to go on.

"Week 21: Well I made it. I was so nervous all last week thinking that this is when we had Gage and lost him. I am so glad to be through. In only 3 more weeks she will be as old as Connor was when he was born. I still get a little scared every time I feel her kicking, like if she tried too hard she might come out. Anyway, I'm seeing my doctor again tomorrow but so far he says everything is great."

I push back from the computer screen and stare again at the name I never knew they had chosen. Suddenly Gage becomes more than a miscarriage, and I realize that, at least to Missy and Charles, Connor was not their first son. In their minds they had already suffered the death of a child, an innocence that had been lost. I remember again Missy's fierce desperation when a year later she had looked at Connor connected to IV drips and a ventilator and monitors that displayed the rapid beating of his heart. He had looked good to her. That was what I had not really understood until now. He had looked like a miracle because he was at least alive. There is nothing we could have said to her, no further hardship that Connor could have suffered, that would have ever made Missy admit that it was time to stop. If he had died, as he came so close to doing over and over again, it would have been with his delicate birdlike ribs cracking as the compressions were pounded down.

I cough to counteract the tightening of my throat and open a soda. There is the sharp sound of escaping air and I wipe absently at the small eruption of fizz that sprays my lap as I scroll further down the page.

"Week 25: Our daughter is now older than Connor was when he was born and she is still safe inside. I know that this time everything will be fine because even if she comes tomorrow we have done all this before. Of course I want her home with me and if she ends up in the hospital for months the way that Connor did, it will be hard to spend so much time with her with Connor to take care of too. But we made it to twenty-five weeks! Smooth sailing from now on."

This is the Missy I remember. Still I cannot really blame her. Like me, she must hear the ringing of the monitor alarms sometimes in the chugging of the dishwasher or the electronic locking of a car door parked just outside on the street.

I continue to sit in front of the computer long after I have finished reading, unable to look away. I do not cry, although it occurs to me. It is not sadness that I experience exactly but instead the dizzying passage of time. I am struck by it all at once and I feel myself reeling. Months have gone by, years even, and I do not know what, if anything, I have actually learned. I can feel the heft of the laryngoscope in one hand, visualize the passage of my ET tube past the winking cords. But still it is a part I am only playing at. It hardly feels real.

In the room next to where I sit, the nurses are changing shift. Greg, with whom I have been working all day, is seated with a young woman with sharp green eyes. He runs down the board on the labor and delivery floor, telling her the ones we are likely to be called to see. Then he briefly gives a report on the two infants strapped into their car seats and attached to oxygen saturation monitors, telling her what time they can be returned to the nursery after ensuring they do not suffocate when seated upright with soft cushioning on all sides.

"Who's on tonight?" the newly arrived nurse asks Greg.

I should turn and introduce myself, let her know that we'll be working together for the next several hours, but I stay as I am. The thought of meeting yet another stranger makes me weary; it has been a long day already and the night will be long as well. I will have to feign confidence and authority, when I want only to sleep. I want to sleep and to have the passing of the hours heal me like it had for

Connor. I want to grow stronger rather than weaker with the shifting of each day. My grandmother would have said I had nothing to worry about. But then she never would acknowledge I was less than perfect, could never see me as I see myself. I think maybe that the blind adulation my grandmother had for me is what it is to really be family. It is the thing about Missy that I had never really understood; Connor would be her perfect child no matter how many scars we laid upon his fragile skin. I am sorry for not having seen this earlier. It would not have changed anything we had done for Connor or said to his family, but it would have changed how I remembered those first days.

From the corner of my eye, I see Greg nod his head in my direction. Even when he has finished speaking, I have to reassure myself that it is not only wishful thinking, that I have heard him right.

"Don't worry. You'll have a good night. She's great. She doesn't even need us there."

I laugh to myself, and this time the tears do come, because it is the sort of thing my grandmother would have liked to hear.

Finding Home

"I promise that it isn't always like this," Christy tells me.

She is beautiful, with a child's face and a sort of guileless enthusiasm that somehow has survived all that she must have seen. I want to believe her, want to put the sort of absolute trust in her that pupils do with their first teacher. That is the sort of devotion Christy should inspire, but I cannot say that I believe her, because I know that the words she means to be so reassuring are not entirely true.

The last time I saw Christy, Max had lay dying, unconscious and with glassy fish eyes that sometimes opened, seeing nothing, not awake enough to even know that he had lost.

It was not only Max I thought of the night before I started on the bone marrow transplant (BMT) service and Oncology. There was Sammy, whose parents had been so much in denial of their daughter's condition that they had continued to torture her with needles and tests and hospitalizations long after any difference could be made. There was Casey, who had lingered on dialysis and a morphine drip until his mother had grasped a yellowed hand that had once belonged to her three-year-old son, pressed her lips against his clammy skin, and decided to let him go. And Molly, face puffy from the steroids and there in all the Christmas photos snapped when we had sung carols in the halls. She had gone home shortly after that day in December, and I, recognizing the girl but not the name, had picked her up when she came into the ER just days before the holiday. She was feverish and neutropenic from the chemotherapy, meaning that she had no power to fight whatever infection it was she had inside. She was sick, I knew, although she didn't look it yet. When she left the ER, the intern I had signed her out to at the end of my overnight shift had checked in on her once more, sending a text message to the resident on the floor with the toddler's most recent (stone-cold) normal vital signs. Molly stopped in radiology for a chest X-ray on her way up to the floor. On any other day, this might not have made a difference. But on that day, by the time she traveled the rest of the way upstairs, she was hypotensive and in need of pressors. She was immediately transferred to the ICU, where she was intubated and on a ventilator for a week before her parents decided to withdraw care.

"Molly went home to die. I hope you know that," one of the oncology fellows, Abby, would later say to me after the flurry of e-mails and meetings that tried in vain to figure out what had gone wrong. "In the end, it wasn't how her family wanted it, but it would have happened no matter what we did."

She is telling me something I already know. Molly was one of those patients for whom, when called to her bedside, it was entirely appropriate to run. It is why, when Molly had arrived in the ER and was sitting quietly in her mother's arm looking tired but not remarkably unwell, she had been watched so carefully through the open door of the exam room, had had her antibiotics started right away. Abby is trying to be reassuring in the same way Christy had been when she tried to convince me that most of the moments in this business of caring for children with cancer were times of success instead of failure.

It is my second day on BMT and I had come in early to review the vital signs and urine output on all of my patients from the day and night before. The fellow who had been on call in the hospital for the service had given me a brief summary of overnight events for all of the kids I had met just one day before. When she finished, I had asked, without guile and without the smallest glimmer of suspicion, "What about Kenny?"

She had not spoken for a moment, tired and in shock.

"Kenny died. I thought you knew."

Relationships in this service, once formed, are written not only in blood but in sweat and tears. Christy had been called at home and she had come in immediately. Jessica, the attending on service, although not Kenny's primary oncologist, had found someone to watch her own daughter and had come in as well. Leslie, the director of the BMT unit, had been on the phone with everyone involved, making sure that they all knew what to do. By that time, Kenny was already dead, but that did not mean it was over. In some ways, it had only just begun. The other families on the floor, even though it had happened behind closed doors and in the middle of the night, knew something terrible had occurred. And Kenny's mother, after making the phone call to her husband, sat waiting in the room with her dead son. Jessica sat with her, in uncomfortable silence, unwilling to leave her completely alone but not able to offer any meaningful solace, maybe because she did not really know the woman, maybe because there was really nothing anyone could say that would have made one bit of difference, that would not have rung hollow and horrible against the tiles spattered with Betadine and blood.

So as much as I want to believe Christy, I know that I cannot. It must be there on my face, in all too plain sight, because she says, "No, really. It isn't like this. I swear."

She speaks as if offering to make a pact, as if spitting on our grubby palms and shaking, or slicing our thumbs and pressing them together, will somehow bring Kenny back.

"This shouldn't have happened," she says firmly. "No one dies pretransplant. He hadn't even really gotten any chemo."

What Christy means is that transplant can kill as surely as the cancers that force children to go through it. After the radiation and the chemo, the body is not left with any way to fight infection. These children die of respiratory infections or from bacteria in their blood. Kenny had not gone through any of this. His immune system was compromised because of his cancer, but it should not have impacted his heart; he had not had any of the medications that are toxic to those muscle cells and are another reason that fighting the cancer can create new problems where before there had been none.

Later that morning, once the sun has come up and the remaining children on the unit have been cared for, we discuss Kenny's case some more. We review the facts, how he had been inexplicably tachycardic for at least a day. That first night, when I had gone home, his heart rate had continued to rise until it was beating faster than a newborn infant's, fluttering over two hundred times in a single minute, and then it had suddenly stopped. We decide that his heart could not have been quite right. Like the other oddities about this child—the way his eyes were set just a little too far apart or the way his muscles were never quite strong enough to keep him sitting upright—there must have been something in the way that his heart was assembled, something perhaps in the proteins that made up the muscle itself, which meant it was destined to fail under the slightest bit of stress. The team would have liked an autopsy, to be able to know for sure, but Kenny's family refuses. They know he had not been born healthy, and they do not want him taken apart like an experiment gone wrong just to give his doctors the answers we could not otherwise have found. It is a kindness, they believe, to spare him this one last abuse, not yet ready to consider that knowing might have given them some solace as well.

This is how it is then—or it is, despite what Christy is saying, the way it feels. Children die. In the whole of the hospital there are beds that are filled with boys and girls who have missing portions of bowel, or brains that cause them to seize, or holes in their hearts. They say that the first thing you must learn in residency is how to walk into a room and recognize whether a child is sick or not sick, whether you have time to think him over or if you need to run. There is another important distinction that can be made just by looking through a child's electronic medical record, and this one is almost as important: if the child was previously healthy or if there has always been something very wrong. You can tell the latter by the myriad of notes from specialists, the discharge documents from prior hospitalizations, the bevy of reports on chest X-rays and CT scans and MRIs. They are different from the children with diarrhea who receive IV fluids on the first day of their admission and then go home again. They have a history that means they are much more likely to break.

When Kenny dies, I am reminded of a lunchtime session that had been dedicated to talking about the ICU. Several times each year, the hour usually reserved for educational conferences is set aside for a session on humanism, on balancing work inside the hospital with the lives we are trying to live outside. Our residency class was divided into groups of six. I found myself sitting with people with whom I was friendly, had sat talking with over beers or cocktails, but with whom I had never actually worked before. We were fed pizza and asked to put words to our emotions, to grapple with the psychological and physical stresses of working on that floor. The facilitators, well-meaning faculty, were strangers we had never met. The conversation moved forward like a secondhand car driven by someone who does not know how to let out the clutch. It was meant to be cathartic, to instill within us, if not answers to our deeper questions, then at least the reassurance that we were not alone in our frustrations, sadness, or fear. We talked for a while, Max was mentioned and remembered by those who knew him, then we fell silent again.

A resident named Colleen said the thing that I remember the

most clearly, perhaps because she had made a habit of saying what she meant in plainspoken terms even in front of large crowds, but more likely because it felt so true.

"It would have been helpful if someone had told us ahead of time that all the Onc kids were going to die."

She said this and my head was not the only one that nodded in affirmation. We each had moments of such helplessness to look back on, it seems, though at the time they had made us feel so terribly alone. Colleen, often blunt and unwavering, did not mean to dismiss or diminish the struggles that children like Max or Sammy or any of the others had been through in the ICU. Neither did she mean to erase the efforts their doctors and nurses had made in hopes of saving them. She just meant that it hurts to watch everything you have done for a patient end in such heartbreak. It hurts to be the only one who did not know it was coming before it finally arrives.

In the end, it was a good session, or as good as such a snippet of time stolen from a hectic day can be. I think about it as I sit alone overnight on the oncology floor, separated from the BMT unit and from Kenny's death by the space of two weeks and two sets of double doors.

The sign-out I get on the evening of that first night on Oncology is that nearly each of the dozen or so patients is holding his or her own. It is not that they are well or that disaster is not waiting to strike in the darkened corner of each room, but they are stably unstable and will probably remain that way for the twelve hours ahead. They all have names and diagnoses I will be able to mumble in my sleep by the close of the week, but for now I keep the folded pages of my sign-out in my back pocket or else tight in one hand and do not put it down. On my feet are another pair of embroidered Chinese slippers that I have bought to replace the faded pair I had worn out during the nearly two years I have been walking these halls. The shoes, stiff in their newness and garishly fuchsia and orange, are a bolder statement than I would have been willing to make when merely an intern. There are moments when I have deserved them, when I have ordered tests decisively and offered explanations to agitated families that calm them without any doubt. But there is also this moment, sitting opposite my classmate Tamara at the wide work table at the center of the doctors' conference room, when the whole night is ahead of me and I do not know what I will need to do.

I am told that I should check in on Harold, a five-year-old boy whose parents are Dominican but who was born in the United States. His leukemia had been treated for nearly a month while he lived in the hospital. Now the number of white blood cells being made by his bone marrow is increasing, and he is nearing the time when he will be allowed to go home. I am meant to check in on Harold because of his breathing, because earlier in the afternoon it was faster than it should be. Over the last hours it had returned to normal and he looked comfortable, but still it was something that could not be explained. The films that had been done of his chest did not show any haziness or opacities that could be called diagnostic, but still he had been started on antibiotics as treatment for a pneumonia.

In the room, Harold is much too small for such an austere name. Even knowing his age, I had expected a pipe and wire-rimmed glasses, a silk smoking jacket, and dark knowing eyes peering out of a bespectacled face. What I find is a thin dark boy in a Power Rangers T-shirt fighting with his brother for the single controller of a video game. Along the far wall, on the other side of Harold's bulky hospital bed, sit a row of older women, a grandmother and two great aunts. Harold's father is a radiology technician, and we talk for a while about the way he had been breathing a few hours before.

"Does he look better to you?" I ask, because it is the parents who are the constant, who see the changes as they come.

His father looks down at his son's chest, at the rate of rise and fall. Harold had lost the battle over the controller and is leaning back in bed, making playful bites at a french fry he is holding just before his lips but without ever eating it.

"I wasn't here before when it was very bad. His mother was." Then, as if an explanation is needed, "She just went downstairs to buy a coffee. She'll be back soon if you need to ask her, but I think that the way he is now looks good."

He is right. Harold is breathing less than twenty times a minute, and his chest wall, when I lift his T-shirt, moves easily without any pulling around the ribs. I do not hear anything but the smooth rush of air as I listen beneath his shoulder blades and clavicles and along the lower part of his back.

I summarize for myself as much as for Harold's father when I say, "The film we did of his chest earlier in the day didn't tell us anything, but he's on antibiotics anyway just to be sure. I just want you to know that if he has another episode where he breathes as fast as he was, then we need to talk about moving him to a different room where it would be easier to get him extra help for his breathing if he were to need it. That would mean moving him over to the ICU. He's looking great right now, so I'm hoping that he won't need it and the antibiotics will catch up with whatever he's got going on, but I just wanted to mention the possibility so that if the move to the ICU does need to happen, it's not unexpected or scary, even though I know we'd rather avoid it if we can."

It is about eight o'clock when I leave Harold's bedside, after meeting his mother and saying goodnight to his dad. I have several pages to return, but I call the ER back first. A page from downstairs can only mean one thing, a new admission, and it is better to not keep them waiting if it can be helped. Coming in is a seventeen-year-old, Trent, who has recently had his left leg removed just above the knee because of an osteosarcoma. His chances are good now that the cancer has been cut off, but the chemotherapy he received in combination with the surgery has left him vulnerable to infection. On this night he has already been seen at another hospital just over an hour away, where he had a fever and was started on antibiotics. It is a straightforward story, but one that would have made the doctors at the outside hospital nervous, knowing they do not have the resources to care for Trent if his condition were to go downhill. So they had transferred Trent to the place where he had first been diagnosed and then had his surgery and where his records are all in the computer for me to review as I write his admission note. I piece together Trent's history as I type, waiting for him to arrive on the floor. He does so quietly. The nurse and I go into his room together to unwrap the bandage above where the knee used to be. The incision looks clean, a thin pink crescent of new flesh covering the muscles and bone underneath. It is not likely that this wound is the source of the fever. I am reassured.

"It looks good," I tell Trent and his mother.

Trent replies, "I haven't seen it yet."

"I used to work in a nursing home," his mother explains, "so I've been changing the dressing."

Trent lifts the disconnected thigh from the bed, a foreshortened arrow pointing up toward the ceiling lights. It swings wildly from side to side and he places it down again.

"We could find a mirror," I offer, looking to his nurse for confirmation that this is indeed possible, and she nods brightly. Trent agrees to look, so the nurse retrieves a mirror from the drawer and angles it below the developing scar for him to see.

"Weird," he says. "It looks really red."

"That's from all the new blood vessels that are helping the skin to grow there," the nurse says. "It will fade over the next few months, but you should be careful not to let it get sunburned. The skin will be delicate for a long time."

She puts the mirror face down on the bedside table and gathers up the ribbon of gauze we had unwound from Trent's leg. Placing a fresh square of heavier packing over the stump, she delicately wraps the long strip around again and again until it is taped into place. It is unnecessary at this stage to prevent infection, since the incision has healed over, but at least it provides a padding while Trent learns to maneuver this partial limb without rubbing it raw.

Back in front of the computer, the ER pages again just as I am putting in orders for Trent's labs and medications. When I call down, I hear about Bryce, who is nine and in remission from a leukemia that was diagnosed one year before. He came into the ER with vomiting, a common complaint as the weather was becoming warmer. His cancer should not have been a factor, because it was meant to be gone, and a quick blood count showed that this was likely still the case. But Bryce also has a blood clot in one of the vessels of his brain that had been discovered after he came in with the worst headache he had ever felt. There was no way to remove the clot. It would not have been worth the risk anyway, since it had not cut off the supply of oxygen to his cortex. There were collateral vessels through which blood could flow. It is not clear, even after much careful review, why this has happened, but the primary goal is to just see that it does not get worse. So Bryce is taking blood thinners twice daily when he comes into the ER. He gets a repeat of the CT that had first showed the filling defect caused by the clotted blood, and this time he has a clot in two of the other vessels on the right side of his head.

It is not something that should have happened in the first place, but it is most definitely not something that is expected given the medication he is on. The ER can tell me only that he is coming in for observation and for some pain medication to relieve the headache he now was admitting that he had. It is a worrisome story because there is no quick test to measure if Bryce is getting worse. By the time the squeeze of his fists grows noticeably weaker or his speech becomes sloppy, the damage will already be done. I can only order the increased dose of blood thinners that has been recommended and hope the night passes without incident while he sleeps.

Before he arrives, though, I am called back into Harold's room, where he is sleeping fitfully and breathing far too fast. The monitor that reports the readings from the circular sensors taped onto his chest only intermittently displays a number that I believe, picking up much of the movement of the boy as he turns from one side to the other. I count out his respirations at 65.

"Do you want me to get the BMT fellow?" the nurse asks.

And I say, "Sure," agreeing easily because I do not know what to do.

Harold had done this earlier and then his breathing had quieted down. Still his oxygen saturation had remained stable. If he was truly decompensating, I would have expected it to drop. I continue to watch Harold breathe. There are faint crackles as I listen over his chest, but they are not nearly as impressive as I would expect from someone breathing this quickly. I order a chest X-ray and ask his nurse to repeat his temperature. When the BMT fellow arrives, I tell him the things that I know about Harold, a story that is incomplete but sufficient for the decisions that must be made.

"What do you think?" he asks me when I have finished.

I pause and glance toward the door.

"Let's step outside," he agrees.

When we are standing outside of the room, he leans his lanky frame against the hallway wall.

"He can't keep doing this and stay here," I say.

"He's on antibiotics?"

"Just since today. Ceftriaxone and vancomycin."

"What about Bactrim?" he asks, wondering if Harold is being covered for PCP, a pneumonia caused by a bacteria that can flourish in anyone who is immunocompromised.

I shake my head.

"He's on atovaquone just for prophylaxis. They talked about switching to treatment dosing of Bactrim today but wanted to wait in case he needs to have a bronch. He was tachypneic this afternoon, but then his respiratory rate normalized, so they decided to wait."

This part of the plan I did not entirely agree with (alone with this sick child overnight), since the safest course of action would have been to give Harold the extra medication. Still, I understood it was not ideal to begin a course of treatment before first obtaining the samples of mucus from his lungs that would be needed for a definitive diagnosis of this illness we were not sure Harold had. If this was not PCP, then to overreact would mean keeping him in the hospital just when (after more than a month spent inside) he was getting ready to go home.

"His sats never dropped?"

"No. He never needed oxygen at all," I tell the BMT fellow. Then, because we are both at a loss of what to say, of how to fit together the pieces of this puzzle that should click neatly in place but somehow refuse to, I say, "It's weird."

"It is weird," the fellow agrees. "When do you want to call the ICU?"

"Now, I think."

He settles back and slides his hips a few inches down the wall, bending both of his long legs so that his scrubs hang straight from the small knobs of his knees.

"I think so, too."

I talk with Anjali, the senior resident in the ICU, when she answers my page and she tells me that she'll come right away. I review Harold's chest X-ray, which is not perfect but still looks much better than the boy it represents. Then I am told that Bryce has arrived on the floor. Walking back out of the work room into the main hall, I pass Anjali.

"I have to see a new kid," I apologize.

"That's fine. I'll find you after I see your other one," she says, meaning Harold.

I am relieved to find Bryce a normal-looking child who is able to answer my questions about his younger sisters without hesitation, who is able to string together the words to tell me about the summer camp he will be attending without a single slip of the tongue. His neurologic exam is entirely unremarkable. I explain to his mother what she has already heard downstairs in the ER and also on his last admission a few months ago. There is nothing we can do except watch him very carefully to make sure he continues to look good.

"Am I going to die?" Bryce asks.

I am startled, both by such candor from a child so young and because I do not know the answer. Even had I had the time to go through all of his records before this first encounter, I would not have felt comfortable interpreting these disparate bits of information. He has cancer, I think, as I look at Bryce from the foot of his bed, and though he is in remission, I have no idea of how long that might last.

"No one is dying tonight," I promise instead, hoping desperately that it is a pledge I will be able to keep.

But Bryce is unsatisfied and holds up his right hand toward me, the fifth finger extended upward into the air.

"Pinky swear?"

I am overwhelmed with the singularity of the moment. I feel the connection between myself and this creature before me, still new and untested, but profound in his depth. This is what they talk about, those physicians who have come to the end of their careers, when they say that it has been fulfilling in a way that no other job can ever be.

I cross to stand just beside him and offer my own pinky, which Bryce links with his own.

"Pinky swear," I nod in encouragement while blinking back ridiculous tears.

In the hall, one of the nurses asks how Bryce is doing. I have an overwhelming urge to tell her what has just happened—the vulnerability, the trust.

"He asked if he was going to die," I say.

She smiles, short brown curls framing her face.

"He always asks that. That's just Bryce. Did he ask you to pinky swear?"

And as quickly as it had come to me, that sense of purpose, of belonging, it has dissipated, leaving behind only the warm suffusion of what there might someday be.

"Hey," Anjali says as she approaches from Harold's room. "We'll take him. Can you write out paper orders?"

She hands me one of the forms still used in the ICU, which had still not yet managed the transition to computerized order entry that the rest of the hospital had undergone. I jot down a transcribed list of Harold's diet and medications and pass it to Anjali just in time as she walks behind the boy's bed when he is wheeled away.

There is a different feel to these nighttime shifts, a sense of separation from the events of the day. I am better rested walking into the hospital each evening than I am when I am expected to work thirty hours straight, but the momentum that carries me through that cycle—the deliberation of rounds and the examination of each patient, the writing of notes and the interpretation of the results of diagnostic tests—is blunted as I walk beneath the dimmed hall lights to crack the door of first one patient's room and then the next. The goal, if all is well (or as well as can be reasonably expected), is to leave these children alone as much as possible. For those who are spending months of their young lives in this strange environment, routines take on an elevated importance. Bedtimes are sacred and sleep should be allowed to continue undisturbed, so there are children I never see during those nights when I move with the shadows, faces I remain unable to connect with their names and conditions despite having committed them to memory. I follow labs and make slight alterations to the infusions that these children receive without ever seeing their open eyes.

Grace is different, though, and I remember her from the first day I came in to meet the patients before my first night of call. It was Tregony, another resident in my class, who had admitted Grace from the ER.

"I thought she was going to die right there in front of me," Tregony had said during the lunchtime meeting when we had talked about Max and Sammy and all the others. My month on oncology had not started, and I did not know Grace yet.

"I don't think I've ever seen anyone look so sick," Tregony told me, shaking her head as she remembered.

Later I had opened Grace's X-rays from that day and had seen what Tregony meant.

What had happened was that Grace started coughing. She still went to school and played with her friends like any other eleven-year-old, but she got tired early and sometimes fell asleep even before she lay down in bed. When the coughing got worse, her parents brought her to their pediatrician, who ordered the first chest X-ray Grace had ever had. The film was not a good one, I think, looking at the scanned-in image on our radiology server, but it is easy enough to see the fluid in her chest. Grace then came to the ER, where they repeated the chest X-ray and called the interventional radiologists to snake thin and pliant pigtail catheters (named for the way they curl inside of you) between Grace's ribs to drain the fluid around her lungs. She was assigned to the pulmonary team because it was not yet clear what was wrong.

When the fluid drained, Grace felt better and stopped coughing. Even before the cytology results from the fluid came back, it was possible to see more clearly on the chest films, once the white of all the liquid was gone, that the bright shadow of her heart was much bigger than it should be. The cancer was the same density as the fat and other tissues that surround the heart. The doctors saw this on the first CT on that same day that the cytology told them it was a malignant neuroblastoma that had been growing inside of Grace's chest. I imagine a surgeon slipping one gloved hand into the very center of this little girl only to have the cancer crumble and ooze at every touch of his instruments, impossible to dissect away. It is inoperable, this infiltrative film of destructive cells, and while the oncologists were consulted and made plans for chemotherapy, it seemed best to let Grace and her family go back home. The fluid that was drained had not come back in the twenty-four hours after the pigtails were taken out, so her parents were told that as long as Grace was not having trouble breathing or lying flat, the hospital was not a place she needed to be.

Tregony is in the ER when Grace comes back, lips wide open as she leans forward and tries to pull air into her lungs. The film that is taken right away shows the fluid has reaccumulated and in fact is worse than it ever was. Her entire chest is white with only two small black domes of air at the apex of each lung. She is taken immediately to an OR, where the surgeons are called to put in chest tubes that have the width of an adult's thumb so that they can drain more quickly than the smaller pigtails. It is immediately clear that until Grace's cancer is treated, she will not be able to go home again.

I meet Grace about two weeks later, after she has been receiving chemotherapy. The drugs that are meant to target the rapidly dividing cancer cells also damage the delicate mucosa of her mouth and nose and impair her ability to heal. Her chest tubes have continued to drain the cancerous effusions, so she is receiving saline and sugar water through her IV, pumped into her veins rapidly in an attempt to keep up with her fluid loss. Because she is putting out so much of this drainage, it leaks around the edges of the tubes, and there are times she sits in wetness, unwilling to allow her mother or her nurses to move her bottom so that it can be dried. The skin over her buttocks is red and looks as though at any moment it might bleed. She does not want to be cleaned or patted dry because of the pain it brings to be touched between her legs and because every small motion pulls at the tubes and she says she can feel them moving inside. From the center of her enormous air-filled mattress, Grace barks orders to her mother to bring ointment or another towel and to put them only where she commands.

Grace is receiving Dilaudid for the pain because the morphine made her itch. It is delivered at the press of a button, in small discreet doses, but it is like dipping a teaspoon in to deflect the water of an oncoming tidal wave. Even after her skin has begun to look much better, she refuses to move.

"I'm worried at how much pain medication she's getting," Grace's father tells me when I am called in on the second evening I am there.

From the beginning of this conversation I recognize that there are things about which we fundamentally disagree. Grace needs more pain medication, not less, because if you are fighting against a disease and have giant hoses stuck into your side, it's unreasonable for people to expect you to endure this torture without some adequate measure of relief. This is not the time to worry about addiction. I also carry with me the very real suspicion that this cancer, unlike so many of the leukemias or lymphomas that are this field's success stories, is not likely to be fixed. Grace may not ever get well or even get better than she is right now. If this turns out to be the case, it is our responsibility to make sure that she remains as comfortable as we can make her, to give this family a quiet unencumbered time in which to say their goodbyes.

I do not say this to Grace's father, for it is not a conversation that he is ready for or one that should be held in the middle of the night with someone he has never met.

Instead, I say, "I understand your concerns. You're right that it's a very strong medication, but I think it's one she needs. She has very good reasons to be in pain. We put two holes somewhere they don't belong and her body is going to react to that."

"She never complained like this before."

On Grace's first films you can see the pigtails winding along the back of her chest wall, no thicker than a drinking straw.

"These chest tubes are much bigger than the ones she had before."

I do not know this man, but I do have the advantage of knowing what has happened before, the conversations that were had, although I was not there to hear them.

"One thing that we often do is give just a little bit of the medicine all of the time," I tell him, pretending that I am not aware that this is a conversation he has already had. "For most patients this actually allows them to push the button less. By not letting the pain ever get too bad, they worry about it less. They stop pushing the button when they are afraid that it might hurt soon and only use the button when it actually already is."

"But she's using more medicine now than right after these tubes were put in," Grace's father protests.

"I know," I say apologetically. "Unfortunately, it's just the way our bodies work. We don't respond to these medicines as strongly after a while. It's the same for everyone. It's not just Grace. It's just the way it is. If you want them to work, you just have to give more."

In her bed Grace is sleeping as we whisper beside her. The hospital gown she wears is untied and lies like a blanket upon her, from underneath each side of which the chest tubes emerge. I bend to look at the fluid accumulated in the containers hooked onto the side rail of the bed, pink tinged and almost unbelievable in its volume. In her left fist is clutched the plastic PCA (patient-controlled analgesia) button. She stirs slightly, without even waking, to press her thumb down to trigger a narcotic dose. It is horrifying to me that she has been so quickly conditioned, a puppy salivating at the first ring of a clanging bell. I place a hand gently on her arm in the lightest of touches, but I do not take the button away. The following night when I return, Grace is on a continuous Dilaudid drip, and she smiles, not broadly or with any spontaneity, but it is a small blessing at least.

For a few days during that month, I go to the clinic just across the road from the main hospital and I follow up with the consult team.

This had been a hard-fought battle, this time carved out of our inpatient responsibilities. Despite the fact that so much of medicine is conducted in outpatient offices, our own schedules did not mirror this. It was on the inpatient teams where we were most needed, providing the hospital with the most potential revenue, and so that is where much of our time was spent. With the consult service, I visit Harold, who is still in the ICU. Since the night I transferred him, he has had the bronchoscopy to diagnose his PCP and is receiving steroids and Bactrim to treat the infection. He is intubated and on a ventilator, having gotten progressively worse since the night I was first on call. Harold's family members sit with him around the bed, stationed between monitors and machinery. They are solid olive-skinned women, quietly issuing prayers from between their broad lips. They wear loose, many-colored cotton dresses and reach hesitant fingers out to wipe the spit dried in the corner of Harold's mouth, careful to not disturb the breathing tube or the strips of tape holding it in place.

Later that day and as if in a different universe, I meet Stuart, who is in the clinic for the first time. I am grateful for these hours spent in the outpatient realm. Despite the two toddlers with recurrent brain tumors, one of them wearing a pink leotard and tutu stretched tight over her steroid-swollen body, it is generally a cheerful place. I walk past one room containing a four-year-old little girl I had last seen on the BMT floor the afternoon I discharged her. I wave and her mother smiles and raises her hand. This is where it really happens, where children who were once dying are told that they are well. I listen to the oncologists' plans for follow-up in six months instead of three or for tapering off the last of a child's meds.

Stuart, two years old and with a slightly pointed chin that predisposes his face to a mischievous grin, is here for his Day One talk. It is the conversation that happens just after a new cancer is diagnosed, when it is decided what will be done, when a family meets the oncologist who will be the primary doctor for their child through the chemotherapy and beyond. But Stuart was diagnosed more than a month before, on a vacation in Louisiana. He was admitted after tests were done to find the reason for his bleeding gums and the bruises on the soft undersides of his thighs. It was during that first ER visit that they discovered the leukemic blasts circulating in his blood, cells that were so numerous that he was not able to produce enough platelets to keep him from bleeding at the slightest touch of the pliant bristles of his toothbrush or his father's hands closing gently around his wrist. Stuart received the first cycles of chemotherapy for his acute myeloid leukemia (AML) in the hospital to which he first was brought and stayed in the ICU only briefly for low blood pressure associated with an infection from a type of bacteria of which I'd never heard.

"What's that?" I had asked the attending, pointing to the bacteria's unpronounceable moniker when I was leafing through Stuart's file.

The attending shrugged: "Something from alligators, maybe?"

We leave it at that, since what matters is the bacteria's sensitivities to antibiotics, and I make a note of the combination of drugs that should be given if Stuart has a fever during the admission he has ahead.

In the exam room, Stuart is bald and unsteady on his feet. He walks the way a ten-month-old does, pulling himself to stand using his father's pant legs and moving from one stationary object to the next. He giggles, but he does not speak.

"He lost a lot of strength when he was in the ICU," his mother explains when she sees that we are watching him move around the small room. "He's only just beginning to walk again."

I bend to hand Stuart a plastic toy figurine that he has dropped just out of reach and he laughs out loud.

"He likes you," his mother says. "He loves girls, the little flirt."

She is pretty, with short blond hair that is economically pulled back into a loose ponytail. She wears a loose-fitting T-shirt and cargo pants that stop midcalf. Her sneakers are trendy and have Velcro straps. I immediately like her, for the casual but tenacious displays of an individuality that is being maintained despite the illness of her only child.

On the floor, after he is admitted, Stuart rides through the halls in a red plastic car. He arranges plates of plastic vegetables and then throws them on the floor. He takes naps during his naptime and he goes to bed at eight. When he has finished his next round of chemotherapy, we perform a repeat bone marrow biopsy that shows his cancer is gone. He is in remission. Even the molecular test that scans for residual disease and will determine what maintenance chemotherapy he will need over the course of many months suggests that Stuart's prognosis is good. In the meantime, Stuart's mother has found out that she is pregnant.

"We always wanted to have kids close together," she says.

I am impressed at how easily she seems to have taken this in stride, thinking forward to a future when Stuart will be healthy and home and ready to be a big brother to the baby she has growing inside. On the surface it looks uncannily like denial, but over the weeks we've spent together I have come to realize that it is something else. Stuart's mother understands that her son's cancer may come back. She also knows that there is nothing she can do besides trusting his doctors to give him the best possible chance that he can have. Her job is not to cure him or to be his physician; it is to be a mother to her son. It is why she continued to allow Stuart to nurse, though the calories he got were negligible. It was about comfort even if it was not important for his nutrition. She could not choose the chemotherapeutic agents he would be given or order the blood tests that frequently needed to be sent. But she could do this still, could cradle him up against her just as she had done on the day when he was born, keeping him close so that they could each feel the beating of the other's heart.

It is only a few days later that I admit a five-year-old girl with

Down syndrome who has just been seen in the ER. Her initial bloodwork shows that she has leukemia. She will need a bone marrow biopsy and other tests before it is clear what kind. As her child and husband sleep, this mother wants to know if all of the progress they have made over the past six months in the girl's language and fine-motor skills will be lost during the long hospitalization that she will face. They are the sort of questions Stuart's mother often had, appropriate and necessary for the family so far into treatment but not for those for whom treatment has not yet begun. This is denial, coming so soon after the little girl's diagnosis, but they are wonderful questions nonetheless. Later, once this mother has moved forward to the place that Stuart's mom now had come to rest, they will be the most important questions of all.

I had been asked many questions during my month on this service, not the least of which had been to pinky swear. And I had been offered the briefest of glimpses into how children and their families were coping with illnesses that would threaten—no matter what the outcomes—to define their lives. I would be moved by each of them. It would never be the other way around. But sitting in the room with that mother and her sleeping child, I have a chance I had never had before. I explain about the occupational and physical therapists who will come to see her daughter every day, the language specialists who will work with her while she cannot be in school. It is reassuring to this woman in a way that nothing else at that moment could have been, to know that whatever tests her daughter will have to undergo, whatever toxic medications she will receive, there remains the understanding that there is so much more to her besides these things and that she is still a little girl.

Walking down the hall, I spin on one heel and stop, uncertain for a moment where I had been headed, what I had strode out of the conference room so determined to do.

"Are you looking for me?"

I laugh, although I know that I shouldn't, because Harold is waving to me from the doors that lead off the floor. It has been about a week since he came back to us from the unit, since he was weaned off the ventilator and has been breathing on his own. He is still being treated for the pneumonia that sent him upstairs, but he is nearing the end of the twenty-one-day course. His cancer is in remission and the medications for this acute illness are ones that his parents could give to him at home. He remains in the hospital because he is deconditioned; after so long lying sedated in bed, he is not able to walk. When he calls out to me, it is from a tricycle given to him by his physical therapist to strengthen his legs. He pushes down on the pedals with bright orange sneakers.

"Did you see my new sneakers?" he asked with unbridled excitement when he put on the sneakers for the first time. He had raised just one toe, unable to lift his foot from the floor.

Now he moves slowly, inching forward, as the pedals are laboriously spun. His legs emerge from the fluorescent Adidas as if they are merely skin stretched over narrow bone. In comparison, the shoes look enormous, appear as if they belong to some older male relative and have been borrowed on a lark.

"I'm not looking for you," I tell Harold. "But I'm very happy to see you. Keep doing your exercises."

I remember then where I had been headed and I take a few steps more to knock on Stuart's door.

"Today's my last day," I say as I wrinkle my nose slightly. "I just wanted to make sure I got a chance to say goodbye before you go outside."

"That's right," Stuart's mother says as she pulls her son to a standing position on the wide bed. "Tomorrow we get all new doctors."

"Not all new," I tell her. "But the residents change. You've got a bunch of great people starting tomorrow."

"Are there any girls?" she asks. "This one isn't happy if there's no one to flirt with."

I smile and reassure her: "There will be several girls for him to choose from."

I will not be at the hospital for the whole of the next month, but I promise to stop by when I return.

"We'll be here," she says with a sardonic smile. I am once more impressed with the way she has taken this life and made it her own.

The walls of the room, where they are not cluttered with medical equipment, are occupied with stacks of toys, molded plastic doorways into fantasy that are each of them labeled in block capital letters written on masking tape. TRUCK, the letters say, or PICNIC BASKET, or FRUIT.

"I'll see you later then," I say.

She smiles and tickles Stuart on his sides.

"What do you think? Can you give her a high-five for the road?"

And he brings down his pale palm with its five perfect fingers to slap resoundingly on my own.

There were times during that month when Grace was not entirely miserable, when her pain was fairly well controlled. Then, she might smile. She might laugh (holding her sides as still as possible) when her father told a joke. Still, no matter which point I choose to leave from, no matter which moment I choose to remember, I know that Grace is dying. There is no way to spin it that will leave it any other way. I am actually surprised to see her name on the board four weeks later when I walk onto the floor. She is no longer my patient, so I ask Aly, one of the new team of residents, where things have come to stand. I know about the CT scan that showed the cancer shrinking slightly but still nestled in all of the nooks and crannies around her heart. I know about the effusion that had built up in the sack her heart rests in, and I had pulled the drain from the hole just to the left of her breastbone when the liquid had been taken off. I had sat up nights turning up her IV fluids and electrolyte replacement to make up for the six liters each day that was pouring out of her chest, and then, only days later, had turned the fluids down when we realized everything that we put in was just coming out again. I know she has had a second round of chemo, based on the marginal success of the first, but after this point I do not know any more.

There is part of me that wishes I could leave it at this point. I cannot picture a homecoming for Grace that will have any honest smiles in it, but I can think of her surrounded by family at least, can imagine her sleeping without pain. Aly pages me: "Grace is going home today." I finish rounding on my own patients and walk over to the oncology floor.

"They found a way for her to go home with the chest tubes," Aly updates me.

"Is she still putting out six liters every day?"

Aly shakes her head. "Only four. But her electrolytes are stable—not normal but stable with the nutrition that she's getting. If we don't send her now, I feel like she'll never go."

I pause for a moment and consider.

"Is she DNR?" I ask.

"I know. I feel like she should be, but no one has had that talk. Her parents just aren't ready."

Before her parents had even known she was sick, Grace's cancer had spread too far. They were still catching up with events that had happened months before, invisible to them, a cellular invasion against which we had no defense.

In her room I smile because I have to, because in such a situation a lie is the least that I can give.

"A little bird told me that you're going home."

And Grace smiles in return.

"Not the red one?" she asks, referring to the brilliant-colored cardinal that lives in the hospital gardens and has two females fighting over him.

"No," I tell her. "One of your doctors told me. What are you going to do that's fun as soon as you get home?"

She cannot move from the bed, but I do not acknowledge that. I ask the question as if she might answer that she is going to ride her bike or jump onto a trampoline. It is a play we are acting out. When Grace turns to her mother with a questioning look, I see that it is a falsehood this woman recognizes as easily as I do.

"You can tell her," she says to reassure her daughter.

And Grace turns back to me and exclaims, "I'm getting a kitten. It's a boy and he's white, but his feet have two big black spots."

For a moment, inexplicably, I am angry instead of touched. I think, "Of course," and I am frustrated by the cliché, knowing that Grace will not be able to drape her arms around the animal's neck for long. Then I remember how her mother had looked at me only seconds before, the hardness about the mouth and just beneath the eyes. I know that she is nearing the close of a journey that will end with her signature at the bottom of a piece of paper that says we do not have to try any longer to save her daughter's life. Because of this, she should be forgiven everything, every small sliver of happiness no matter how inadequate that she tries to bring into the days or weeks that they have left to share.

"Do you know what you're going to name him?" I ask.

"His name is Sox with an *x*."

And I say, "I think that's a perfect name."

A week later, Aly pages again. This time it says, "Grace is back. CT much worse," but I cannot come right away. When I do enter the room, the smile is harder to summon. There is nothing I can say that will not ring hollow and will not sound more like an insult than a comfort. Grace's mother lifts a hand to wave but looks too tired to speak. In the bed, Grace appears unchanged. Her cheeks are still swollen and both nostrils flare with each shallow breath. Looking down at her, I feel suddenly what it would be like to drown, slowly and agonizingly, as she will surely do. My throat catches and I cannot breathe, my own impotence as heavy on my chest as the fluid within Grace is heavy on hers. I stand frozen for too long a time, but neither Grace nor her mother notice. Animated figures dance across the television screen and Grace reflexively pushes the button to deliver a dose of Dilaudid before reaching out to pull a stuffed animal in closer to fit under her arm. The room feels empty despite being cramped with too much furniture. My skin is cold as I finally manage to take in a lungful of air. As much as I resent it, I realize as I stand there that this job could not be half as wonderful—there could be no Harolds or Stuarts to bask in the joy of—without it being exactly this hard.

I force myself to smile as I say, "Tell me about Sox," and move forward into a chair.

There are places that it is possible to disconnect from and walk away, but this floor is not one of them. Perhaps it is because the balance that Christy had spoken of all those weeks before, the happy fairy-tale ending that exists for those who are cured, is not one that we get to see. We are shown glimpses, only, during the afternoons we are allowed off the inpatient floor and into the clinic, but it is hardly enough. So instead I am left to imagine what comes after, to offer my own version of what should be.

Harold will stay well. He will be carried up the steps into his apartment. Someday, after a few more weeks of therapy, he will walk out again and play on the swing set across the street. I roll this scene backward and forward in my mind until I believe it might be true. There is no reason for it not to be. I do not have to hope for it against all odds, because the odds are on his side. For Stuart, too, there will be a homecoming at a place where the scrub pine gives way to sand, where he will be able to grow and play. His chances are not as good as Harold's, because AML is a more difficult entity than

ALL, but he achieved remission quickly and his repeat bone marrow was clean. I cling to these possibilities and I try to make them true so that when I smile my goodbye to Stuart or push Harold's tricycle down the hall, my expression at least is not a lie. I know this is what Christy had tried to give me: the knowledge that even though not every child I care for will be able to get better, not every interaction is a falsehood, not every reassurance is a deceit.

What the Voices Tell Us

There is a day as our last year approaches when they find us coverage in the hospital. Several times a year the residents are excused from clinical responsibility to assemble elsewhere—at the Lovejoys' beach house in Annisquam or at an outdoor conference center with a high ropes course and pulley system that allows our program director to be foisted, protesting, up into the air. Back in the hospital, fellows and attending physicians cover the services they usually just oversee, responsible once again for the sort of paperwork they had been more than happy to leave behind, spurred on by the shrill refrain of pagers going off with demands for stat orders for Tylenol or Mylicon or Desitin for a troublesome diaper rash. In the evening, despite their best and valiant efforts, discharge paperwork will remain unsigned and the tidy patient lists used for sign-out will have dissolved into disarray, leaving the on-call interns and residents to spend the next fourteen hours putting things in order all over again.

So it is not entirely a relief when our day-long senior orientation arrives and we find ourselves in a downtown hotel conference room with puce-colored carpets, faux chandeliers, and coarsely faded drapes. Those of us who had been on call the night prior let our chins fall forward onto weary chests. During this hiatus (a space of only ten hours) will be compressed all that we need to know to run the inpatient teams on which, until now, we had been only the cogs. We are transitioning from scut monkeys mindlessly moving from one urgent task immediately onto the next to something more evolved—the people who must have answers and not only questions. We have learned how to succinctly shuffle paperwork from place to place, to update sign-outs, to get patients efficiently into and out of our doors.

Now, over stale Danishes and burned coffee, they intend to infuse us with vision, show us the big picture. They intend to teach us leadership. They mean to transform us, if we have not already learned how to fill this role by trial and error, into teachers. Standing before us, they underline the importance of making interns feel welcome and supported, of creating an atmosphere of synergy and teamwork. They highlight the need to encourage each rotating medical student to develop his or her own fund of clinical knowledge, of correcting mistakes privately while publicly lauding the things that have been gotten right. In small group sessions the chief residents and program directors scrawl key ideas in brightly colored markers. They write on giant pads of paper of the sort we used to read song lyrics from on lazy afternoons at summer camp. They condense it down, neatly and with bullet points, as if anything in life can be that simple, let alone something that is this big. They give lectures on respect and inspiration, never once acknowledging how difficult it is for those skills to ever really be taught.

They offer these various pearls of wisdom as if they are prescription drugs, to be taken at such and such a time and on an empty stomach, after which they will certainly work all the intended miracles: "Remember how overwhelmed you felt that first day that you started. When you want to offer instruction, use the feedback sandwich. Come up with one or two nice things to say to the intern or student you need to take aside to talk to. Then transition to the thing they need to work on—it's not that they are doing something wrong. Make them see it as an opportunity to just do it even better. Then throw another compliment their way to end on a positive note, just like putting another slice of bread on top."

So, later, when it is my turn, I say, "This is a new team and I just want to say first how excited I am to work with and get to know you all."

I sit at the head of a cramped and cluttered table at the City Hospital. Our work area is small and without windows, natural light as always being reserved for the patient rooms. Two walls are lined with computers that routinely freeze and delete complicated narcotic orders before they can be signed. High shelves boast an odd mix of pediatric textbooks and journals interspersed with stashes of bottled soda and single-serving pretzels, caffeine and salt being main staples of late nights. The lights above sizzle and cast greenish yellow shadows in the hollow crescents beneath sleep-deprived eyes. The interns should still be fresh, but they do not look it. Only a handful of weeks into the year, the schedule has begun to take its toll. They flip through the stacks of papers before them, pausing to underline an increase in respiratory rate or drop in oxygen saturation, running down the list of patients whom they will soon have to present without faltering and with a confidence they surely do not feel.

At home each of them likely has unpacked boxes. They have tapestries from trips in Europe or South America that they have yet to hang. On their bureaus are arranged framed pictures of the parents and grandparents who gathered at their medical school graduations, aging loved ones whom they had hugged tightly and promised: "Don't worry—we'll talk all the time." They have already grown used to overflowing inboxes, voice mails, and promises to stay in touch they will not know how to keep. They look too young to be here, even though there is not much difference in our ages, and I have a sudden urge to shield them from what the following months will bring.

At orientation, Vinny Chiang, the director of inpatient medicine at Children's, had told us, "It is important to begin with expectations, both so you can congratulate someone for meeting them, but also so when you need to give constructive feedback, you have an easy reference point from which to start."

So I say, "We'll round with the nurses in this room, go through the patients and their plans. Then we'll do walk rounds as a small group with the on-call resident. We'll see a few of the kids who are likely to change the most in the next twenty-four hours. The goal is to finish by nine o'clock. If we can do that, it will give most of you enough time to do some work and see your patients and hopefully still get to our teaching conference morning report."

Just as they told us to do during orientation, I describe the big picture—how each day should ideally have time enough for work as well as for learning—all the while knowing that the interns will have to put blinders on just to survive. They will hunker down to get through their notes and the writing of new orders, and it will be entirely up to me to make sure that it actually happens this way. In reality, rounds will often run slightly over and we will have spent the majority of the morning holed up behind closed doors, logging onto sluggish computers, reviewing the morning's labs, and leaving parents to wonder where exactly their doctors actually are.

Acknowledging that this system was less than perfect, a few times each year efforts were made to get back to family-centered rounds, an ideal that all too often does not find a place in the rushed schedules that we keep. On family-centered rounds we would move from patient room to patient room in a slow progression down the hall. The interns and medical students would take turns presenting the infant's or child's history, with the parents and the patient's nurse included in the circle, each having their chance to offer observations and to be a part of deciding on a plan. I understand the appeal of such a system. If I were a parent, I would want to see the time and effort that was being put into my child's care. But there are thirty patients on the floor. If there were fewer beds (as in the ICU), then we would have hours to spend on every patient; we could see to it that every family felt reassured that the care we were giving to their own child was the most important thing in the world. But in an overburdened system, walk rounds have largely been determined to be unwieldy. It had been tried many times before my own internship and several times during and several more times since. But these walk rounds invariably stretched to noon, hours during which medication orders were not written promptly and discharge paperwork was left undone. They were at best a nice gesture, but one that is not as important as the other less visible and necessary vigilances that will see their sons and daughters day by day becoming well.

Now I am aware of the clock and our absence from these patients' rooms during the first few hours of each day in a way I had never been before. I try to move rounds forward, call in the nurses, and let the interns tell me what they would like to do. Each patient is (for them) still a mysterious and individual person on whom they are reporting, and there are times that things move slowly. They have not yet garnered enough experience to neatly slip each newcomer like an index card into the slot that most accurately describes why the child is here. It is a trick we learn only over time and by painful repetition, but it is one I have come to rely on, each time seeing in my mind a picture of the first child I cared for who bore that diagnosis—bronchiolitis or gastroenteritis or diabetic ketoacidosis (DKA)—and therefore knowing what we will likely have to do. The four-year-old girl in this room is an asthmatic; the teenage boy in that bed is a sickler in VOC (vaso-occlusive crisis). Occasionally we are chastised for this sort of reduction, this boiling down of sugar water into hard candy. It takes something away, people have argued, to label others this way. Solzhenitsyn warned against such treatment in *The Cancer Ward.* Whereas there are real shortcomings in medicine, this is not always one of them. It is a fine line but not a slippery slope, and it can be walked along if it is done with the utmost care. Ultimately there is a difference between the shorthand we employ to describe our patients, to transfer essential information from one caregiver to the next, and the cold perversity with which it has sometimes been equated. The truth is that the faster I can safely describe a patient to my colleagues, the more time I will have to spend in that patient's room.

This time comes after rounds have finished. I walk with Courtney, the other supervising resident. A gaggle of medical students and at least one intern follow. We examine the children who have cellulitis and outline in pen the discoloration of each skin infection so that when the antibiotics penetrate and begin to take effect, we can measure the resolute retreat in its distance from the border that has been marked. We listen to each of the wheezers and watch the rise and fall of their thin chests.

In one room we find a dark-skinned boy of about eleven. He is breathing quickly as he takes in the nebulized albuterol through his open lips. The boy's mother sits beside him with the morning paper. Their television, unlike the others we have seen that morning, is tuned to CNN. While his breathing improves, the medical students cluster around him and press stethoscopes lightly against his chest. They train their ears to pick out the racing heart sounds layered beneath the louder wheezes, the whistle that is the escaping of trapped air. The boy removes his face mask as we prepare to leave. He leans back in bed to watch the news.

"He looks good, doesn't he?" I remark and nod upward to where the bulky television set is fastened to the wall.

The boy nods and continues watching Barack Obama answer questions shot at him by reporters along the campaign trail.

"Do you think you'll ever be on TV?"

Again he nods and this time he looks at me.

"I'm going to be president someday," he says.

On some mornings, there is a period of blessed but unnerving quiet. If the admitting pager remains silent and no one on the floor is deteriorating, there is a time when I have nothing that I need to do. The interns are making phone calls. They are writing notes. They bustle about from room to room wrapped in an air of muted frenzy that gives the impression of great importance, and I am almost jealous as they pass me by. They are performing tasks that I have become good at, that are familiar, but they are tasks that are no longer mine.

"It's not your job anymore to oversee every little detail," both Vinny and our program director, Bob Vinci, tell us at orientation. "You have to think about the floor as a whole and you have to trust your team. Keep an eye open. Make sure things are getting done. But don't make them feel like you are looking over their shoulders, just that you are there to give whatever help they need. It's hard, but try to let them ask for it."

It is a difficult one, this transition, and it is one only the best teachers ever fully make. It requires a confidence in one's own skill that I am still lacking, an ability to deftly select from all of the stories, the vignettes, that one from which something dangerous has been omitted. It is a way of listening for an absence rather than its reverse—so that like a line of poetry with an uneven meter, it sounds so obviously unfinished that it reflexively signals the additional investigation that must be done. It is a talent that I lack, so there are certain patients I worry over and whom I make sure to see early on each day.

Samantha is admitted to the floor only days after she had last been sent home. This last admission had been to the ICU, a small unit that is comprised of only five or six beds unlike the several floors of critical care rooms we sometimes work in at Children's just across town. Although impaired developmentally from the moment of her birth, before this last ICU admission Samantha had always breathed in and out on her own. Then there was a stretch of time during which her heart had stopped beating, when it had to be restarted with paddles slapped down onto her bare chest. This was the moment that divided her short life in two. There were the five years that came before her pulse was lost and chest compressions were started, and there was everything that would come after—the weeks when she would be on a ventilator and the day the trach would be inserted in the hollow above her collarbone. She does not move or speak or even meet my eyes on the day we meet. Reading through her chart, that is not a change from how she was before.

Her tiny frame is too small for the oversized hospital bed she lies in. She is covered with handmade quilts while her mother rubs buttermilk into each of her limp, motionless hands. Samantha has always been fed through a G-tube. Her mother has always massaged her legs, braided her hair, and stuffed pillows first on one side and then the other to keep her from getting deep bedsores. It helps that she's tiny, can easily be picked up, and her skin is beautiful. I comment on this as I examine her, because Stella should get whatever small rewards can be dispensed for taking care of such a complicated girl.

When Samantha vomits, we stop her feeds. When she spikes a temperature and her heart races, we send blood cultures and give empiric antibiotics that she probably does not really need.

"We're still getting to know her," I explain to her mother, a dark woman with a quiet face that never betrays impatience even when this is surely what she feels. "She's probably going to be different than she was before. You'll have to help us recognize the ways that she has changed."

The truth is that Samantha's brain, though never normal, now does not have the ability to regulate itself. These rises in her temperature probably do not represent infection in the way that they once would have done. It is the same with her rapid breathing, her widely fluctuating blood pressure, her alternately racing or plodding heart.

A Haitian ensemble chants "Alleluia" from a dented battery-powered tape player. When the song reaches the end, it automatically flips over and the tape begins again. It is a vigil Stella is keeping, sitting beside her daughter's bed, one she has kept for the past six years, so she spends it chatting infrequently with visitors and more often on the telephone. She can care for Samantha herself. She bathes the girl with warm washcloths. She connects the tubing to her G-tube and hangs the bags of formula for her feeds. It is as if she is indulging us when we enter to perform our exams. She seems happy, contented. She asks only when she can take Samantha home. I think that perhaps she wants nothing more than for things to stay the same, as she has known them. In many ways they always will, because Samantha will never really grow any older than she is. So Stella can afford to be as patient as she seems, biding time until we release Samantha, but still refusing many of the additional diagnostic tests that we suggest. In the weeks that she is with us, we never actually determine the reason she had so much trouble being fed.

When Samantha is no longer vomiting, we decide to release her. We have not gotten any answers, but even so, there is nothing more that we can do in the hospital that Stella cannot do at home. Because she is so complicated, I read through her medication list myself before I submit her discharge paperwork to print.

I am on call with Blaire, the one intern from our group of four who has had the most difficulty with this year. Having struggled during earlier rotations, she had faced the frustration of her colleagues at things left undone or presentations stumbled over during rounds. Courtney and I had even sat down before the month began to discuss how we would keep the peace if things escalated as they had before, how to avoid the tears in the ladies' room and the snarky comments made just within Blaire's hearing and then—boldly but cruelly—right to her face. Luckily, the pace on the floor had been steady but not too overwhelming, and the workload had thus far been fairly easy to split.

If I were a better teacher, I would make Blaire send Samantha home. One of the skills she had been found lacking during earlier months was cross-covering during her nights on call those patients cared for by other interns during the day. Overnight she would be called on to make decisions about patients she might never have met. She sat quietly during afternoon sign-out and made notes on her patient list, but when it came to anticipating the needs of those patients with whom she was less familiar, Blaire sometimes let things slide. The details of sending a child as complicated as Samantha off the floor—the prescriptions for her special G-tube feeds, the home nursing approval, and the volume of each and every liquid medication—were things I knew I had to double-check myself. As I run through the list one final time, Blaire sits at the computer next to me putting in basic orders on a new admission. I know that when the nurses poke their heads into the workroom to ask the occasional question, this probably looks like seamless teamwork, that we have decided to divide and conquer, our hands moving over each of our keyboards in some wordless synchronized dance. I type a quick addition into Samantha's discharge note and hit the icon to print. Blaire passes a hand over her hair, rearranging the dark strands and tucking them back underneath the clip from which they have escaped. She punches in her password to sign the orders she has entered and then turns to me.

"I think I'm going to go lie down for a little while."

I am caught off guard, so I do not immediately object. When I had been in the ICU at Children's the year before, I had been similarly tongue-tied when challenged by one of the nurses about a conversation with an angry mother. I had not been certain enough in that moment of disagreement where the authority should lie. Now I know with clarity that it is my job to tell Blaire that she has responsibilities that distinctly preclude sleep. On her last rotation Blaire was rumored to have remained in her call room for the duration of the night when a patient stroked and was rushed to the ICU. Then it had been three or four in the morning, and however inexcusable it was to have been absent from such an event, it was not entirely clear in the retelling that when the first page had remained unanswered, her senior resident had actually bothered to have Blaire paged again. This time it is only eight-thirty in the evening and Samantha, our last planned discharge of the day, has not even gone home.

"Don't wait for the end of the month to begin giving feedback," Vinny Chiang had told us. "You need to be comfortable giving it all along. Otherwise the interns won't have a chance to work on getting better."

Instead, I say, "I'll page you when something happens," knowing that I am being weak instead of kind but that it will not matter for too long. Blaire is unlikely to be able to escape for more than a few minutes this early in the night.

Early though it is, I appreciate that she might actually be tired. I know how it can hurt just to blink sometimes, your eyes desiccated from thirty hours of being open and exposed only to stale recycled air. I understand the need to carve out even just five or ten minutes to lean your head against a pillow, to bend down and take off your socks. Call is not something I have taken to well. I would be lying if I told Blaire that she will grow accustomed to the hours or days lost sleeping in recovery from a long shift, or if I did not admit that when I looked at my call schedule each and every month, I was counting down as well. If I had met her on a bus or at a party, we might have spoken like friends and I would have been able to commiserate. I would have been able to agree when she tells me that it isn't fair (because it isn't), but these are not the roles that we are cast in. Watching the door close after Blaire, I feel the missed opportunity and realize how much less I am than the role model Blaire needs me to be.

There is a reason giving feedback was such a large part of our orientation and had been touched on practically every time the administration talked with us as a group. It is not something we residents do well. Our program director, Bob Vinci, might say it is because pediatricians are nice people, but that is a feedback sandwich, too. The truth is we are uncomfortable passing judgment on another person whose shoes we have just barely traded in. It is not an easy job the interns have. It is not possible to do it well or to even feel adequate at the task. It is a struggle always as much as it is a reward. And while I am nervous about making Blaire uncomfortable (or more accurately, making myself uncomfortable), it is something I know I have to face.

I page her not ten minutes later when the next call from the ER comes through. The patient downstairs is straightforward, another asthmatic, and I consider whether it would be easier to just admit this patient myself. It will be faster certainly, and I am not quite ready to speak to Blaire. But paging her is the right thing to do, so I force my fingers to tap out her pager number to initiate the call. She returns to the harsh lighting of the workroom and her eyes are already bleary. I wonder if it is possible that she had actually fallen asleep in such a short time. I never would have been able to drift off that quickly, but that is because I am a worrier. Even with the lights out, I run through everything that can go wrong, the labs that will be sent at four a.m., what I hope or fear they will show. I make mental lists of the tasks that are still undone. Blaire, in contrast, seems to have the uncanny ability to turn that part of her mind completely off. It will serve her well later on, once she is able to judge when things are truly under control. But this is not a point she has reached yet. As I typed Blaire's pager number into the system, I remembered again what Steffie had told me at the beginning: "You will not sleep at first because you are too busy. And even when your work is done, you shouldn't sleep because you don't know when it is safe." So I had gone to my call room only on those nights when Rishi or some other senior had expressly told me to go lie down.

"You've got to be kidding!" Blaire exclaims as soon as the door swings open. "That was only ten minutes."

It is ten more minutes of quiet than I have had myself, but I do not need to bicker. In the other corner of the room, one of the medical students works on his presentation for the next day and I know I cannot say anything that I do not want him to overhear. I consider the best way to go on. It would draw even more attention to pull Blaire outside the room to the hall where the nurses congregate and there would be an audience there as well. Still uncertain exactly how I want this to go, I choose something easy to begin and accept that this will be only the first conversation of the many it will take to cover all the things I will need to say.

"Can I give you some feedback?" is too abrupt of a beginning and sets, I think, the wrong sort of tone.

Instead, I say, "There's an asthmatic downstairs. It should be easy."

"I'm so sick of new admissions," Blaire says, and I know that even with all the other things she needs to work on, this is where we need to begin.

She is tired and she does not want to be here. In this she is not alone.

"They're definitely tiring," I agree, even though she has had only four that day. "But we're doing a good job of getting through them. Soon you'll be supervising admissions, which in some ways will be easier. But you should keep in mind that when you are leading the team, it will be your job to motivate your interns and get them through the night. You won't be able to complain when new admissions get signed out."

I am so concerned that I am handling this poorly that at the end I cannot think of another positive slice of bread to finish the sandwich with. I pause. When I still come up with nothing, I wait for her reaction.

"I know," Blaire tells me. "I wouldn't complain to anyone else. It's just I feel comfortable around you."

This is nice, but it is also entirely beside the point. Part of both of our jobs is to act as mentors for the medical student, neglected and working on his notes for the coming day, and she is not doing that. I repeat my point to drive it home. For the rest of the night, she accepts new admissions without comment, which is a small victory at least. After midnight, as is customary, I admit the patients myself. Blaire sleeps. The following day and home in my own bed, I, too, sleep, but not before a fretful hour of contemplating her next feedback sandwich and what I will choose to say.

I escape to the PICU (pediatric intensive care unit) for a half hour or so on some of the nights when Blaire and I take call. I reason that it is important that she learn self-motivation, but in reality I need a chance to vent. Blaire has a habit of entering orders but delaying admission notes until the following morning just before rounds. She leaves things half done and takes breaks in the middle of a complicated order set to call her boyfriend and request dinner from some restaurant that she is craving, which he will then pick up and deliver. Such a piecemeal approach to each and every task is not my style, and I do not think that she will find it workable when she moves on to other, harder rotations. I recognize that at this point it is her choice; still, it is difficult to be in such a small room with her and not feel that I should offer constant commentary on how she is managing her time. My own work I can complete from any of the hospital computers, so I swipe my ID over the electronic lock to the double PICU doors as a portal for a brief escape.

My classmate Lara, with only one patient in the PICU to care for, is checking her Facebook page when I pull up a rolling chair and sit beside her. The PICU nurses sit at their own computers just outside the door to this small office and seem to be shopping at Overstock.com.

"How's the floor?" Lara asks me as I prop my feet up on a stool.

"Steady, but not too bad," I tell her. "How's it going here?"

"Just one asthmatic," she responds. "He's spaced, but I promise not to send him out to you overnight. We obviously have plenty of open beds."

Lara's blonde hair falls in gentle waves around her face. She had been a teacher before coming to medicine and she has a level lilting voice that would have been calming even in the most chaotic classroom. I am thinking about this when I notice the ultrasound picture on the computer screen.

"Who's pregnant?"

"Brie," she tells me, referring to another resident in our class. "She's having twins."

"Twins? Seriously? What is it with our class?"

Andy and his wife, Gina, had just had a pair of girls, Molly and Avery, the year before. A second set of twins seemed to be fairly remarkable.

"I know," says Lara.

"Do you know how far along she is?"

"About twelve weeks, I think."

I count off the months quickly in my head and realize when she will be due.

"What did Susan say?" I ask with just a hint of dread.

Susan is the administrator in charge of making the schedules for all 120 residents. She does not especially welcome having to integrate maternity leave into this already complicated grid. It is an unspoken rule that children should not be conceived after the month of May, when the following year's rotations and vacation assignments come out, and up through September, as any pregnancy begun during this time would necessitate a difficult schedule switch.

"She said: 'I'll add you to my list.'"

"What does that mean?" I ask Lara.

"Apparently, Brie makes number three."

"You mean two other people are pregnant? In our class?"

Lara shrugs: "I don't know what class. But it can't be an intern. No one would do that."

I agree that it seems impossible that an intern, so new to residency and with approximately one hundred on-call days ahead, would have chosen to complicate things further by starting a pregnancy this early on. So we pull up the residency website and click through to the page that has the names and pictures of our class. Slowly we scroll down, crossing people off the potential list.

"I saw her out drinking just last week," Lara says, pointing to one of our colleagues who had signed on for three more years of a rheumatology fellowship when this year was done.

We quickly eliminate people on the basis of alcohol consumption or comments that they've recently made, laughing as we go. It is silly and we know it. Still, we are not the only ones who have gotten hold of the rumor. A little more than a week later, I mention to Neil what Lara and I had done and the progress we made since that night in further narrowing it down. Neil, too, it turns out, has also been part of such a discussion.

"We decided it was you," he tells me.

"It's not," I reply, honored somehow to have been considered.

"But we decided," he repeats playfully.

"Well, in that case, I'll have to get to work."

I am not pregnant and there is no chance that I will be anytime soon. Daryl is desperate for a baby, but I have had to tell him no. After having the same conversation several times, I made him a spreadsheet with my upcoming residency requirements, highlighting the ones notorious for being especially difficult and during which I could not imagine being pregnant. The hardest rotations stretched up to the end of the year and would be followed by that no-fly zone where becoming pregnant not only meant risking Susan's pained expression—the thin line of her mouth indicating the impossibility of the miracles you were asking her to perform—but ruining one of your colleague's schedules if you did have to arrange a trade. In the end, Daryl had given up asking and instead got paired up by Big Brother Little Brother with a twelve-year-old named Peter who was at times even more mature than he.

On one of the nights I am not in the hospital, an older teenage boy is admitted from the ER. About a month before, Harry had been to his pediatrician's office complaining of a stuffy nose. He was having difficulty smelling things. The young man's exam was normal apart from the clear discharge visible in both of his nostrils. His doctor had prescribed some nasal steroids, which he used to relieve the congestion. His smell returned but only temporarily. For the past week, Harry had been having difficulty smelling things again. He finally comes to the ER because of a headache that will not go away. He has tried Tylenol and ibuprofen. He may well have wished he could try a stronger medicine, but his parole officer would have found this out on his next scheduled urine screen. In the ER, they want to give him morphine. He worries that if he agrees, he will be made to return to prison, so the ER staff has him pee in a cup and they document the negative urine tox before giving him the drugs. They also call radiology to arrange for an emergent MRI, which is usually difficult to get quickly. It is sometime after midnight. His headache, although improving as the morphine takes effect, is not the sort of headache a teenager should have. Radiology immediately bumps the other cases from the scanner and moves Harry to the top of the list.

The tumor sits against the bone in the place where the olfactory nerves leave the skull. The mass, either because it is pressing against these stringlike fibers or because it has consumed them, is the reason he cannot smell. The collection of unwanted tissue seen on the MRI measures several centimeters across. Later, when they get the CT scan to look at that area of skull with better resolution, they see the cancer eroding into the bone. By the time Harry is admitted to the floor, the neurosurgeons have reviewed his films and the ENTs (ear, nose, and throat doctors) have seen him. He is scheduled for a biopsy of the tissue to be performed in the ENT clinic by reaching up through his nose. The neurosurgeons, pending a definitive tissue diagnosis, will likely then go in as well.

On the floor, Harry is in the second bed in a semiprivate room. He has the window, but it looks out onto concrete rooftops with no view of trees or other green. In the bed that is between Harry and the hall is another teenager, this one on the surgical service. He has been involved in a high-speed car crash after threatening a girlfriend with an unloaded gun. Her brothers had tried to run him down in their own vehicle. As he accelerated toward the highway, his car clipped a mailbox and he spun out of control. His femur was broken and his tibia as well, and the leg is encased in an external fixation device. From all angles there are metal skewers impaled down to the bone. His family moves into and out of the room, arguing in Spanish, their voices pouring out along the hall. Harry's only company during this first part of the day are the flocks of subspecialists that bring their residents, their fellows, and their medical students in to perform unnecessary neurological exams. I watch this foot traffic. It is like watching spectators tramping to a circus or a sideshow. A group of more than half a dozen leaves the room, their white coats trailing, and we page the oncology service again.

Unlike at Children's, where there is an oncology consult service that oversees the workup of any new cancer diagnosis, here it is something that happens so rarely the protocol is not really known. Phillipa, in practice mostly a hematologist but also an oncologist by training, should have been called when Harry was admitted. Instead, we call her during rounds, at which point five hours have already gone by. When Phillipa arrives, the ENTs, neurologists, and neurosurgeons are all involved but directionless, with no clear point person running the show. This is not something that affects Harry's biopsy or his access to pain control, but still it is a process that feels disjointed, lacking the neat packaging that would have been provided across town with both compassion and finesse.

"He needs to be transferred," we whisper between us, assuming the barrier is political, that either the ENTs or neurosurgeons will selfishly want to keep such an interesting patient here.

"It's not that simple," Stacey explains. One of the chief residents, she is also acting as our attending on the floor. "Phillipa will advocate for that if she thinks it's best. She's done a great job of that in the past. But he's nineteen. He has a criminal record. It's kind of a fuzzy area. Children's wouldn't know what to do with him."

This is likely a completely accurate, if unfortunate, statement. During Harry's short stay in the hospital, the pediatric social worker talks to his parole officer multiple times a day. She faxes the tox screen from the ER and updates him on the medications Harry needs to be receiving. She smooths ruffled feathers calmly and quickly because these are all things she has done before. But this is not the only thing keeping Harry here. It is also, I am soon to learn, the question of just what the tumor is. The pathology report is still pending after Harry returns from his biopsy, and it will be pending for at least several days as the cells soak up some stains but not others and the pathologists cut thin slices to set upon their slides. It is only when a diagnosis is made that we will know if Harry needs immediate neurosurgical intervention or if treatment with radiation or chemotherapy is first called for instead.

It is late in the day when Harry, nineteen and no longer a minor, finally calls his father. Legally an adult, it is his choice to wait. We had been able to do no more than encourage, to intermittently pester. His mother had died of lung cancer the year before, Harry had explained, and he did not want to worry his dad unnecessarily until he had more to tell. But it is not right that he is alone, the onslaught of visitors not there to reassure or console but rather to examine him briefly only to turn and go.

"Harry's father wants to talk to someone," his nurse comes into the workroom to say.

By the time this happens, Phillipa is long gone for the day. There is an intern on call with me, but we are all that remains of the team. I look around at the empty room and then back at her.

"What am I supposed to say?" I ask.

The nurse shrugs helplessly.

"I was only told that he was here."

At Children's, it is called a Day One talk. Because it is so important, it is something I would never be allowed to do. As a resident working in three different hospitals, I cannot hope to be there for the test results, the decisions about chemotherapy. The person who walks into the room to tell a family that their child has cancer should be a doctor the family will see again. But even at Children's this does not always happen. Brian, one of the Children's Heme-Onc fellows, had once been coerced into coming to dinner to be set up with one of my friends. Both he and she were aware that they were meant to meet but, less than impressed by my attempt at playing matchmaker, they spent most of the meal talking to other guests. As Daryl ran back into the kitchen to plate out the third course, Brian told me one of his patients had just died.

"They decided to withdraw care. After that, it happened quickly, but I didn't know. I only found out afterward, and by that time, the family had already left the ICU."

This was a child who, after diagnosis, had seen another fellow in the clinic. There were other residents, fellows, and attendings who cared for the little girl on the oncology floor and, at the end, in the ICU. But it was Brian whom the girl's father would point to and say, "That's my daughter's doctor," because it was Brian who had been there on that first day.

There was no snappy metaphor recited during our orientation to prepare me for this day. They might have said, "Be prepared for anything," or "Expect the unexpected." Either would have been good advice, but they would not be adequate for the depth of the task that I now had ahead.

I push my way through the crowd that has gathered around Harry's neighbor, brushing past plump arms and wide floral skirts to finally reach his bed. His father sits in one chair and his sister in another. They both wear jeans and T-shirts that are as faded as the hospital gown Harry is in.

"Every patient, every family that you meet will have different expectations," is what they should have said. "Every situation will call for you to take on a different role. The trick is to walk into a room and know instinctively just what kind of doctor they need you to be."

I introduce myself to the rugged man with the silver crew cut as one of the doctors taking care of his son. I start by asking what Harry has told him about what has been happening and he tells me that it is not much. So I tell him that because of Harry's symptoms—the headache and problems with smell—an MRI had been done. I tell him that there is a tumor nestled against the inside of the boy's skull. I tell him that because of where the mass lies (I avoid the word *lucky*), the ENTs had been able to get a piece of tissue without Harry having to undergo surgery.

I finish by saying, "There's a lot we still don't know. And I'm sorry that I'm not the expert on what to expect. You'll certainly get a chance to talk to those other doctors as we start to know more. But what I can tell you is that based on what the biopsy results tell us, we'll be able to know what kind of tumor it is that Harry has. From there we'll be able to decide whether the best thing to do is surgery to take the tumor out, or if it would be better to give radiation or chemotherapy before any surgery is done."

There is a moment of quiet. On the other side of the thin curtain separating the room's two beds and only inches away from the small circle we have made, an aunt or cousin says something in Spanish. There is laughter. The curtain billows and then hangs still. I pretend not to notice. Harry should have privacy, but there is nothing I can do.

"So it might not be cancer?" Harry's father asks, and I see the hope in the space between us like some rare and precious bird that I know I will have to kill.

"No, it's definitely cancer," I say so that there is no more confusion. As gently as I can, I continue, "But there are many different kinds of cancer and we don't know yet what kind Harry has."

"That's why they did the biopsy to be able to look at the tissue," Harry's father says tentatively.

"That's exactly right," I agree.

"And that's why we're waiting for that report."

"From the pathologist," I confirm. "But Harry doesn't need to be in the hospital while we wait for that. We need to observe him overnight and tomorrow he can go home. You'll certainly be able to talk to the oncologist, the cancer specialist, before he goes anywhere. And we'll set him up with all of his doctor appointments and make sure you have all the phone numbers to call any time of the day if you end up having other questions. This is a hard time. I know it's scary and the waiting is difficult. But if there's not a real reason for him to be here, I think it will be better for Harry, better for all of you, to not have to be in the hospital."

"Sure." Harry's father nods his head in affirmation. "We just want to get him home."

Harry goes home and comes back several days later to be admitted to the adult ICU. In that unit, while they decide whether he is stable for brain surgery, he is cared for by a whole new group of doctors whom he has never met. They are concerned about the progression of new right arm and leg weakness, symptoms that had worsened gradually over the course of nearly a day and that he had been tempted to ignore. By the time his father makes it to the hospital, Harry has had a stroke with such severe bleeding that he is paralyzed.

But before that, when hope still sits between us wrapped in a box tied with silver and gold thread, we talk until all Harry's and his father's questions are answered. When we are finished, his father thanks me so profusely that I feel even more guilty, knowing that it should have been someone else they remember from that day, hoping that I have at least come close to being the kind of doctor they wanted me to be.

Just after this month ends, Daryl and I host a dinner to celebrate the completion of this difficult rotation and I invite the entire team. Only Erik and Courtney come with their spouses; the rest of the group are busy with call or out-of-town visiting girlfriends or just escaping from the city. This sort of underwhelming attendance is not surprising. Rather than cancel, we invite a hodgepodge of other friends to round out the crowd. Brian comes over again, but this time I do not bother searching for a single friend with whom to set him up, since he really is in no need of help. Merielle, in my original class at medical school and having just moved to the city, is free as well. She has already finished her residency in obstetrics and gynecology and is an attending at one of the city's smaller hospitals. Without the time I took away from medicine to study at Oxford, I would not have met Daryl, but still I am jealous of Merielle's new job and the fact that she is done with her training and starting something new.

In the kitchen, Daryl is furiously chopping vegetables to go with the roast chicken, a dish that should have been in the oven long before the guests arrived. It is a hurried affair, this dinner, with both of us arriving home from work later than we had planned. Still, as the night progresses and the food emerges in stages, I begin to enjoy myself. Even though the entire team is not assembled, those of us who are there talk about how the month has gone. It is a tradition, the time-out for reflection, that should be practiced more.

Erik, the only one of the interns to make it, offers up several stories of his own, coolly mentioning how we had chosen one medication instead of another or had ordered a certain diagnostic test. Some of the words he utters so casually were not even in his vocabulary four weeks before.

"Try to see yourselves the way the interns see you," Bob Vinci would tell our class on many occasions. "You don't realize how much you've really learned until you do."

I realize that though I had been selfishly relieved that Blaire was unable to come, it would have been good for her to be here. She would have had stories of her own to tell and we would have had the time, for once, to really listen.

When my parents stop by after their drive in from the airport, there are still a handful of people there. We have dessert and conversation continues.

"I love that Merielle is here," my mother whispers. "It's important to keep in touch with the people who really know you. Even when everything else has changed around you, friends should stay the same."

At some point, my mother sneaks out of the living room and starts doing the dishes. We discover her only after most of the guests have left and she refuses to stop. Daryl and I join her in scraping cold pasta into the garbage and organizing leftovers in plastic containers. Gradually, the countertops are uncovered and the last of the plates are slid into the dishwasher.

We sink into the couch. The cats, encouraged by the newfound quiet, emerge from the bedroom and find their way into our laps. The living area is still strewn with cloth napkins and empty wine glasses. We will tackle them in the morning. For now it is enough to simply sit.

I realize then what I should have told Blaire but never knew how. I should have said that these years are difficult, but that they should not be wished away. I had been more guilty than anyone of crossing off calendar days when each in-house call was done. I crossed off days and weeks and months and then years, all the while thinking that it was what must be endured before the sweet return of all that would come after. I was counting down to a time when I would not spend whole days cooped up in the hospital without ever seeing the sun, but I was also counting up to a time when I would feel that I had become the doctor that this training was supposed to make me. It was a nebulous thing, this promise of calm and perpetual assurance, and I was only slowly realizing that it was a myth. It was not a single point in time or a rigid destination but a series of stepping stones scattered upon a grassy hill. The path to the knoll would never lead straight up and no two paths would be the same. Erik had reached and stood upon the first of these and Blaire had reached a few herself. There would be other, stronger versions of ourselves ready to see the next patient, to deal with the next moment of crisis, but the doctors that we were in each of those first steps were just as much of an accomplishment as the finished product would be.

Sitting with my family, I know that while I had been counting down, my life had been happening around me. I had not always noticed, so wrapped up was I in the sleep I was not getting or the patients we would not save, but still it was there in the candles burned down to the wick and the glasses emptied of their wine. It was there and it took only a few hours basking in the murmur of voices and in pleasant company to feel fresh again.

The Graduating Class of 2009

I am sitting in radiology on a morning of my last year of residency while the residents and attending review the cases from earlier in the day. I am only half paying attention, but even so I recognize the scans before the CT has fully loaded. I have seen those same white strands of malignancy that are infiltrating her lungs, have seen the bulk of the tumor surrounding her heart, wrapping around the pulmonary arteries and the aorta in a lethal embrace. Even before I see the high-up slices that include her chest tubes, I know that it is Grace. She is still alive, which is something, but it is obvious even to me that she is getting much worse.

"I don't know why they bother," the attending radiologist says, too dismissively I think, although his voice is not at all unkind, "if they've decided to withdraw care."

The small group of radiologists clustered in front of the display station smile as they flip through the studies, safely removed from the children and the pain that they represent. On their screens patients are reduced to black-and-white images. One resident carefully inspects a two-dimensional portrait of a child with a badly broken wrist or fractured rib. Another laughs in between reading plain films that are normal and another that shows a pneumonia, the treatment of which will mean an inpatient hospital stay. The radiologists make throw-away comments about their own lives as they go through the day, and I realize that although they are also physicians, we do not have the same job. There is a distance between this floor and the ones on which the children I know come to stay. It is the brief thirty-second elevator ride to emerge seven floors above, where the rooms have windows painted with snowflakes or shamrocks or colored leaves depending on the month. And it is the presence of those children they are looking at in their pictures—the sound of crying or laughter even from behind closed doors—that is the constant reminder that there is no room for uncertainty in this business of medicine where there is no possibility that anything can ever be known for sure.

Still, though I have a more colorful picture of these children than the images the radiologists have before them—pictures that will never capture the moment when pouting lips break forth into a smile—my actual knowledge of them is only slightly more informed. In the images that flash before us, there are glimpses of time as it is passing, snapshots of what happens when our patients are outside our walls. As often as I wonder what is happening to each of them, young boys and girls with whom I have spent long and painful weeks, intense periods of both mourning and the burgeoning of hope, when they pass through the large revolving doors to exit the lobby, I do not know to what sort of lives they have gone. I have no knowledge of the picnics or play dates, the days they will feel sick or the weeks when they will be entirely well. They disappear, and as curious as I may be I know it is better if they do not return.

The portraits that I paint are incomplete and probably grossly inaccurate. They exaggerate the smaller details to which I have been privy, ignore the larger parts of their histories of which I am unaware. I like to think of Connor sitting in the yard beside his father or of Muffinball being pushed in a stroller while Kay goes out to buy milk. And I like to think of Grace sleeping with Sox at her side. I think these things, all the while knowing that I will be forever ignorant of the lives they actually are living outside of the hospital in rooms where I will never go. It is a comfort to me to imagine the good days they will have. I choose a color—red—for the knapsack that will be tossed casually over one thin shoulder minutes before rushing to the bus. Out shopping, I rest my eyes on a pair of patent leather tap shoes that I know the nine-year-old girl with cystic fibrosis I discharged two days ago would adore. I do not linger, do not even reach out to touch them, but almost without thinking I find myself moving my lips to soundlessly say her name.

More than two years into my marriage, there are times when I have the same feeling about my own life that I do when thinking of Grace or Aban or Max. Unlike the outside world, where I too often feel almost like a stranger, the hospital is real. The hospital is the place where you must keep moving, always learning, the place that drives you forward to keep working no matter how little sleep you've had. At home, where sleep is a possibility, I escape to bed long before Daryl is finished with his day. Though we both wish it were different, Daryl's protests are ones that I can ignore, so I am usually dreaming to the quiet background of the television as Jon Stewart wraps up and hands off his viewers to Colbert. In the morning, when Daryl rolls over to hit the snooze button on his alarm, I am already gone. Even during the few hours of the week when we inhabit the same space, we are still missing each other. My absence is more than simply from want of energy, lack of sleep, my brutal schedule. I realize that there is something that has been missing from this routine and these priorities that I have set and (this far in) I begin to fear that it has not simply been misplaced for a time but instead has been absent from my life all along.

"How did I get here?" I often thought. It was not a question about geographic location exactly but something bigger. I cannot find the words to ask the thing I really mean.

It was hard at times to shake the feeling that I was drifting, although it would not have looked that way on paper. My two years at Oxford read like the same sort of résumé padding I had always abhorred. I had gone there not for the extra line on my CV or even for the degree; I was desperate for my life to begin before I disappeared into residency. I had not known in college in any concrete sense what it was that I should become, only that I wanted to be exceptional, to live a life less ordinary. I had moved to England because it was a different path from the one that was expected, and because I hoped that the dust of ages would soak into my skin. There was brilliance there, echoing against the cold stone floors, but it would never be my own.

It would not be enough, I felt at times, to be a doctor. It was not enough to simply endure the passing of the days, the endless stream of the sick or injured in whose crowded company I sometimes felt as anonymous as they. I had delayed residency for the two years that I lived in England in the same way that I now put off starting a family, because both internship and parenthood seemed irrevocable, high impenetrable barriers that marked endings rather than the beginnings that they should be.

"We can do this," Lara had said partway through our senior year, sitting in the PICU at the city hospital. "I just don't know how."

Lara had spent part of her honeymoon working in Lesotho, something I would never have offered to do. She had worked in South America and spoke Spanish. She was a careful and caring pediatrician, but she did not know where she would be when residency ended. We were all looking forward to that next stretch of years and realizing that it was hard upon us. There were decisions to be made and they were not as obvious as we had expected them to be. Lara wanted to work internationally, but for a pediatrician married to an internist, there were no jobs that paid. There was no way to disappear into the jungle and not default on student loans at the same time.

For Lara and for myself, the future was not at all clear-cut. Sitting in the PICU, reminiscing about how our residency applications had boasted that we intended to someday work internationally, we can think of very few role models to choose from. There is Paul Farmer, who had written books, won awards, and graced the pages of magazines. His home was Haiti, Paris, Cambridge, and everywhere in between. For long stretches, he saw his family infrequently or not at all. Lara and I have to agree that this is not a pinnacle of success we really want to attain. We say it sheepishly and then more boldly, daring the other to disagree or contradict. It is a weakness, we had come to believe, although it had not been said outright, to give in to wanting family at the expense of our careers.

"You'll figure it out," the program's directors said to us at that same orientation that was meant to prepare us for our senior year.

They wanted for us to be leaders in our fields. To achieve this in cardiology or oncology, the path was straightforward and well trod. There would be a fellowship and time spent in clinical research or in a lab.

"We can have both," Lara tells me, making her voice at the same time firm and cheerful, but I am not so sure.

I have not spent any time abroad during residency. I have barely traveled outside the city and cannot pretend to be the same person I was when my residency application was filled out. But still I wonder again if what I am missing can be found only somewhere else. I imagine how wonderful it would be if there were places and entire groups of people in need of something—what, exactly, I could not say—that I alone could give.

"I'm still working on stopping torture." My childhood friend Nathaniel is working for Physicians for Human Rights and he tells me this over the phone as I walk home from work in that first month of my internship when so much of my time was spent trying to keep a premature infant named Connor alive. "What have you been up to?"

And as simply as that, it suddenly seems not enough, the long hours I have spent making changes to ventilator settings or following up on labs. It is not nearly enough because not any of it really is mine. I cannot boast responsibility or accomplishment because there is so much I still do not understand.

It is possible that all this is at least a part of the reason that as I begin to move closer to the end of residency, I board a plane bound for New York, and then another bound for Brussels, and finally a flight to Monrovia, Liberia, where I have agreed to spend the month working on their pediatrics ward. I wish I could pretend it was with an openness of heart and singleness of purpose with which I set forth on this trip, that at the outset I am under no delusion about the magnitude of my own importance in a country with such overwhelming need. I am a doctor, a person with a certain set of skills, but there is no guarantee that they are skills for which there is actually a want.

I had been to conferences on international health and the inappropriateness of certain foreign gifts. Then there had been slide shows with pictures of infants baking in isolettes that had been donated to places without the electricity to run their temperature and oxygen control, the sun shining through the thick curved plastic walls and concentrating the heat there, onto the tiny bodies within. So I knew, in theory, that things do not always go as planned, that entire highways have been paved with good intentions only to find the road should have gone to the left instead of the right. But despite all this, I had a buried if nebulous desire to arrive and quickly become utterly indisposable, to find that finally I was special in the way I had always hoped I'd be.

So perhaps it was partly because of Nathaniel that I got on the plane, because I wanted in that pause that comes between the courses of a good dinner to have something impressive to say. But it is also because Natalie (who had introduced Daryl and me) flew to be at our wedding from Kinshasa in the DRC (Democratic Republic of the Congo), bringing us a carved marriage cup to mark the day. And it is because Emily, who spoke to her mother every day that we lived together at Princeton, somehow managed to move her life to Vientiane while Ellen walked to the market in Namaacha for bagias every week for more than two years. It is because Christine, Princeton valedictorian and gifted musician and physicist, had looked at me one night as we sat in her company's penthouse apartment less than a block from Times Square and said, "I feel like I should be doing something more important with my life. You and Natalie are doing so much good." And just as I had gone to medical school only a few short years after she had turned to me in our freshman physics class and said, "If you were a pediatrician, I would bring my kids to you," I get on the plane because I so desperately wanted to prove her impression of me can still be true. They are a difficult group, these friends, to ever really feel that I deserve.

My bags do not make the last leg of the journey with me, so I have only my laptop when I step out of the plane onto the tarmac. In Brussels, I was promised that they would follow on the next flight into the country, more than twenty-four hours later, and it is unclear how I will arrange to pick them up. I have no idea, in fact, of how I myself will make the hour-long journey into the city, no certainty at all that there will be a card with my name written on it when I emerge empty-handed from the baggage claim.

"No bags?" the customs' officer asks. I can do nothing more than shrug.

"Lost," I tell him.

His face is not reassuring; it is, in point of fact, dismissive. He has already forgotten me and is looking past my head.

"It happens," is all he says.

I fold the yellow carbon copy of the form I filled out to report the missing bags, place it in my pocket, and step outside. The evening light holds a coolness that is not present in the air, which is close around me, moving warm fingers down the base of my spine to settle in the press of fabric where my trousers hang on my hips. I am already hot and must blink a few times before I adjust to the way the light bounces off the white concrete buildings and rises in waves from the black asphalt. Then I see my name before me, written in a crooked hand on a limp placard, held out in offering but noncommittally, as a salesperson might hold forth a sweater she has already decided you will not buy.

I am not sure to whom I am speaking when I point to the sign and then to my own chest to indicate that it is me whom he is waiting for. There is a Dr. Dennis, the director of the hospital, with whom I have been in brief and somewhat intermittent contact. It is possible that he himself has come to fetch me. I am afraid that I will blunder into insult if I do not behave as though it might be him. But nothing more is revealed as the man lowers the sign and turns to indicate the direction in which we must walk to find the car. Another man steps forward, his thin frame inadequate to the task of filling out the loose white cotton shirt he is wearing. He gestures to my bag and I hand it to him, wondering if this might be another of the entourage, a doctor or other hospital personnel. I am confused when we reach the modestly sized SUV and this second man places my carry-on into the backseat and makes no move himself to get into the car. I climb into the front seat and only belatedly realize that some sort of tip is expected, but I have nothing except twenty-dollar bills, and this would be too much. I do not, in this country largely without ATMs and where credit cards are worth only the plastic they are made from, have any cash to spare. The car pulls away to leave him standing there, not angry as he might have chosen to be at that moment but quietly resigned.

The road is smooth and straight, only two lanes but freshly

paved, and we move quickly as we leave the airport, the horn sounding frequently to warn those standing on either side of the road of our coming. The land we are passing through is lush, vivid with the many different shades of green that are long grasses, broad-leafed palms, and shrubs. In the gullies along either side of the road, women are walking, balancing baskets on their heads; children are standing with their hands squarely on their hips and their hips thrust before them; men idle on folding chairs clustered around radios, leaning closer to catch a few notes amid the static pouring forth. The men do not look up as we fly past and the women do not pause in their graceful shuffle. Only the children turn their heads to watch as we approach and pivot on one heel to follow our path until we are gone.

We are going relatively quickly, passing slower-moving cars as we come upon them. Then we stop; the road ahead is empty and the landscape to both the right and left is unbroken by a single building. There is a faded sign placed by the road some fifty feet ahead, an advertisement featuring a cartoon drawing of a young boy holding a can of soda out in our direction. I feel within me the first stirrings of alarm at this unexpected stop, imagining ski masks and machine guns appearing suddenly against the windows, but from where? There is no place in the scrub on either side of us in which to hide. After a moment of stillness, the car lumbers slowly forward and the front wheels thump down the six-inch step-off in the pavement, and we accelerate again. I had not seen the ledge, not from afar, not when we were right up upon it—this break in the smooth ribbon of road before us. From any sort of distance it was not visible. "You are wondering how I can see," Dr. Dennis says to me the following night in his car as we return to the airport to fetch my missing bags. Rather than assure me that he can see just fine despite the utter darkness into which we are plunging, he adds, "I know these roads."

We drive perhaps another thirty minutes through lush countryside before we stop again. By then the lean-tos have gradually been replaced by squat cement buildings clustered close together.

Traffic has slowed and we roll to a stop behind a battered white truck with the letters *UN* stenciled amateurishly on both doors. I wonder if it is really a United Nations vehicle at all, with this oddly inept claim to belonging, or if it is some sort of front for drug lords or diamond smugglers or other unspeakable force. I will continue to wonder about the validity of this authority here, an organization for which I in theory have much respect, each time I walk past the crumbling UN buildings on my way to the hospital, where the young people within seem to be playing at being soldiers much like children on summer holidays might build a fort and sit looking out from within.

To the right of this truck is a stream of people, and it is this crowd of bodies the cars have become mired in. At first I believe we are witnessing the end of the workday or a busload of travelers deposited at some station up ahead. Groups of teenage boys walk in loose clusters, letting the occasional fist swing out to thump solidly on the hood of some anonymous vehicle as they walk by. Pregnant women move somewhat more slowly, in short measured steps, their bellies full and wrapped tight in patterned fabric or peaking shyly from beneath a short cotton tee. Several school-age children expertly carry coolers between them, their tiny hands sharing the handles and somehow managing to negotiate the load without tripping over their partners' sandaled feet.

"Where are they coming from?" I ask Alvin, the driver whose name I learn only later.

"The football match," he tells me and wags a finger at the windshield to indicate. "The football stadium is just there."

"Who was playing?"

"Liberia and Ghana," he says. "A big match."

"Do you know who won?" I ask, although I realize that the lack of jubilation from the scene beyond the window should tell me which team did not.

Alvin shrugs and this time uses one finger to indicate the radio, which for the whole of our drive has produced mostly white noise: "I have been trying to listen."

It is an hour at least before the stadium comes into view and longer before we are moving at a normal speed. By the time we reach the JFK Medical Center campus, dusk has long given way to full dark. Dr. Dennis meets us outside of the emergency room entrance and extends his hand.

"I am sorry for all of the chaos, but we have been very busy here. There are ten dead already from the football game and we just had to put chest tubes in two more."

I learn that there had been a press of ticket holders at the stadium entrance and some undefined structure, above or below, had given way. People had been trampled and crushed, lungs had collapsed and spleens ruptured, and the doctors at the country's leading hospital had been unable to fully repair the damage that had been done. I think about the exodus through which I had just come and realize that it is possible that the screams of the injured could have been absorbed completely by the roar of the crowd, entirely unnoticed by those who were within. I realize also that there was a time when the thought would have saddened me, but now I am hardly wounded by it at all.

"It's lucky that the game was a draw," Dr. Dennis would say later. "There would have been more dead if we had lost or we had won."

The hospital itself, JFK Medical Center in Monrovia, is a shell of the institution it used to be. In this country of riches—it is not just the diamonds, but the land itself, fertile in rubber and sugarcane in all seasons and with easy access to the coast—there had once been a medical community that served not only its own people but those of neighboring countries as well. JFK had been the place people traveled to in order to be seen by specialists. After more than two decades of war, most of the physicians had fled the country or been killed. The hospital that had once been the flagship of Liberia's medical system is only the shattered remains of what had been. The low-lying structures are crumbling even after the repairs that made them usable again—repairs that replaced the missing or leaky roofs but not the light fixtures, that mended most of a staircase but not the handrail running alongside. Bare wires emerge from holes at odd places in the walls, tumbling out in their many-colored bundles with the occasional glint of copper.

The maternity hospital, next door to the main building, stands waiting for money from Japan to resurrect more working OR space. A large sign boasts the relationship between the Liberian government and its Friendship Maternity Hospital and the Japan International Cooperation Agency from whom the initial funds for reconstruction had almost magically materialized. No one I speak with has much idea what this agency actually is. Still, generous though they had been, this initial investment was not nearly enough. The roof on this large edifice has yet to be replaced. During the heavy rains, water leaks down through the stained square ceiling tiles high above the main ramp between the ground floor and the second level, or else blows in to douse this slick incline through windows that have no glass. The inside walls are painted the sort of blue found on the bottoms of swimming pools. The color is garish and slightly revolting without the softening distance of water in between.

Within the squat sprawling structure of the main hospital, the pediatrics ward is a series of three cramped adjoining rooms and one larger open bay. In the main room, wire or string has been stretched to support partially inflated balloons, limp rubber and cellophane stamped with Christmas reindeer or Pokémon figures that are meant to distract the children but that are simply attracting dust. A small red plush bear has been similarly suspended and gives the impression that it has been ensnared by some predator. Below this strange assemblage of decorations, the rows of metal cribs are lined up along each wall with only the space of a few feet in between.

This room is filled with bodies, but it is almost silent; even the children are oddly still. Around us the air is hot and oppressive and the dingy sheets draped on the occupied cribs are damp even to light touch. The thin curtains featuring endless recitations of Jerry chasing Tom, or the other way around, hang high along the pink painted walls and block not only the air but the view over the rooftops and down to the sea. Mothers sit in uncomfortably molded plastic chairs imprinted with the incongruous reminder "God Loves You" or curl their long bodies around their infants, knees tucked high to fit within the cribs' rusting metal bars.

Having arrived finally on the pediatrics unit, it is still unclear to me what my job is meant to be. I am meant, in part, to assess the educational needs of the medical students and residents so that the curriculum can be strengthened by those who would come after me. It was an ambitious project, one that was not yet entirely off the ground.

So during my first day on rounds, I mainly observe and concentrate on the unpleasant sensation of my white coat hanging across my shoulders and over my back, where sweat beads are actually forming with enough rapidity to make a quickly flowing stream in the hollow over my spine. The patients are presented by the four medical students and overseen by the two pediatric residents, women who are easily five or ten years older than I am but who had only just managed to graduate from medical school because classes were suspended so frequently during the war. These women, with about the same clinical training I myself had upon graduation from medical school, had offered to take over supervision of the pediatrics ward because there was no one else who was willing to.

The presentations of each child are detailed but rambling. It is difficult to understand from the narrations just what has been done: "This is D.S., a two-year-old Liberian male, who presented to the ER with a history of fever for five days and cough. . . . He was brought to the ER by his mother and an impression of severe malaria was made. . . . He breastfed exclusively until two months of age and then sugar water was added. . . . His mother is unemployed and his father sells scrap metal. . . . This morning I encountered a well-nourished male child lying in bed, sleeping, in no apparent painful or respiratory distress. . . . The abdomen was soft and symmetric with no organ enlargement. . . . Examination of the groin revealed normal external male genitalia with testes descended bilaterally; foreskin was intact and retractable. . . . He has received two quinine infusions. . . . We will continue current management."

It is possible that I am confused only because I do not know what current management should be. I have never seen malaria. I have no knowledge of the shaking fevers that mostly come at night, the small body prostrate, the lips refusing to part for food. I do not know about the headaches or the vomiting, the frequent bowel movements or the seizures that may be triggered when the parasites have reached the brain. All these symptoms and their treatments are new to me, but they are something I would quickly come to know the rhythm of, as the story is repeated alongside each crib in our circuit around the room.

It is not only the particulars of these tropical diseases that I am unaccustomed to; there is an undercurrent of disorganization that I had never encountered in my training. Rounds move slowly, painfully, as extraneous details are elaborated on and relevant clinical information is too often missed. At the close of each patient presentation, the cumbersome papers stapled into manila folders that serve as charts are handed by the medical students to either Dr. Nuta or Dr. Andrews for review. As they write a hurried signature, we are already moving on. There is something strange about the process. It is not only that this shuffle of paperwork and vital signs and treatment courses is not as well lit or precise or air-conditioned as rounds at home tend to be. There is something larger that is missing, but I cannot at first see what it might be.

It is only after several days that I finally pinpoint the cause of my concern. On rounds that morning, we move from the patient in bed 7 to the patient in bed 9. Bed 8, which had housed a malnourished child who had been placed on oxygen ("Why the new oxygen need?" I had challenged the students, "What was the insult to his lungs?" but had never gotten a satisfactory response), was no longer there. We move past the bed and pause only to look back.

"What happened?" I ask.

Dr. Nuta shrugs, "He expired."

She says this as if it is the kernel of truth buried inside any such story, because children die when there are not enough resources to save them. How he died, what was done for him in the last minute, what things changed to make him appear very sick indeed instead of merely terribly ill—these are not details she offers.

I know that I have not seen the things she has and it is not to challenge her that I continue this line of questioning. I simply need to learn how things here work.

"Who gets called at night?" I prod as gently as I know how, because I know that none of this is actually her fault. She cannot be present in the hospital twenty-four hours a day.

Her shoulders lift and fall again and the answer is essentially the same.

"The intern should get called," she says.

Whether the intern was called or not, whether that first-year doctor covering the entire hospital even arrived on the floor before the youngster let the final breath pass from his lungs, she does not know and has not been told. At Children's, there would have been at least five doctors present to witness any death, after which the entire hospital course would have been dissected to ensure that no mistakes were made. In jarring contrast, it seems that here, because there is so little that we can do, no one feels responsible at all. And this is what is so loudly absent, screaming so insistently and with such a volume that it reverberates from the horrible pink walls, and I am amazed I could not decipher it before. Culpability is not the kindest word to use, but it is one that fits. I carry this knowledge with me like a painful blister on the sole of my left foot, almost worse than the death itself, but I say nothing because there is really nothing to say.

"His Spot was positive and so was his mother's, but she left before she could be told," Dr. Nuta says in a tone as defeated as the final chorus in a Greek tragedy. I realize that *Spot* is their code for HIV.

The following morning we round on a new patient, admitted with a complaint of several days of fever and rapid breathing almost since his birth. The medical student, Trokon, focuses on the fever, explaining the quinine infusion that has been started. Listening, I nod and agree that this medication for malaria, in a country where the parasite is so rampant, is the appropriate course even without any diagnostic tests to confirm. We will treat this infection, I think, and mentally take that problem and set it to the side. Much more troubling is the fact that the child is so severely malnourished despite being breastfed regularly, and at six months he cannot yet sit up.

"Why is he breathing fast?" I ask Trokon when he has finished presenting.

He lifts the boy's chart a little closer to his chest as if for protection or simply for the pause the small movement allows him. "The fever might make him breathe quickly, or a pneumonia."

"But mom told you that he has been breathing quickly all his life. She also said that the baby gets plenty to eat, but he's very wasted. You should make sure you are thinking about other things that might increase his caloric needs, like a metabolic problem or some kind of congenital heart disease."

I say this because it is a good teaching point but without any clear notion that it might actually be true. But when I lean down and place my stethoscope on the thin chest, I hear a roar of blood in the space between valves closing that should be reserved for silence. There is nothing subtle about this finding. Such a prominent murmur should have been picked up on even the most cursory of exams.

This is clearly the reason the boy cannot grow, the hole in between the walls of his heart making it all the more difficult to keep oxygen flowing to all the places it must.

"He needs an O_2 sat and a chest X-ray, and someone needs to try to get a blood pressure reading from all four of his arms and legs," I say in one breath, speaking quickly as if to make up for the time we have already wasted.

Trokon is jotting notes in the patient's chart for these orders while the other students lean over the chest to listen, each in turn.

Their eyes light up as they say, "I hear it." And I think to myself, "I truly hope so," since this is the sort of finding that should be hard to miss. I am frustrated that the presentation of his physical exam, like that of all the patients on this ward, had managed to be so tedious, to include such a vast amount of information (the presence of his foreskin, the fact that he has hair on his head), while completely overlooking the one pertinent physical finding that will in all likelihood mean that this baby (like the absent infant in bed 8) will not get to grow up.

"Can he get an echo?" I ask, wondering how we are to get a picture of the walls and tiny valves that make up his heart, which is the first thing we must do if there is any possibility of repair.

"It is not something that can happen quickly," Dr. Andrews says, almost defensively, although I had certainly not meant to cause offense. "He will need to go to Mercy Ship."

There are many things this hospital is lacking. There is no microbiology lab to send samples for culture. The X-rays are hazy and difficult to read, and there are days when there simply is no film to shoot the pictures on. Each afternoon the power goes out. The city current is stopped and the hospital generator is meant to seamlessly kick in. The reality is that the power goes out several times each afternoon and the windowless clinic falls, without warning, into utter dark. We remain motionless in the cramped space with too many sharp corners or precariously situated paperwork.

A voice in the blackness says, "This is ridiculous," and another answers immediately, "This is Liberia."

When the lights fail to return, cell phones are fished out of pockets and held close to prescription papers, the faint and sickly glow of the screens providing just enough guidance to scrawl orders for quinine and iron tablets. But it is worse for those in the operating theater, who can do nothing but watch the reserve of energy in the anesthesia machines wind down slowly to its end.

There would be no way to run a ventilator outside these operating theaters for more than a few hours or any of the other respiratory assist devices I had come to take for granted during my training in the States. Technology has no place here, at least not yet. There are things that JFK is in want of, and it is a want that is visible in the angle of the physician's jaw as he writes yet another quinine prescription for a child with a negative malaria smear and a worrisome history of shaking and tactile fever, his temperature never verified because no family in this country has a thermometer in their home. It is visible in the set of a mother's shoulders as she lifts her infant onto her hip in that moment of uncertainty when the medical student finishes examining her son but has not formally dismissed them, signs his note, and moves on to the next chart.

There is a weight, a sense of harassment, in each of these moments between physician and family, because in each of them is the enormity of all that they are doing and the even more overwhelming enormity of all that cannot be done.

Back in the States, a hospital is like an enormous organism, with systems and subsystems that are essential to seeing the patients who come through its doors get well again. The doctors and students here should have all of the things I have so often taken for granted. I dream for them a PCR machine, a thousand sterile lumbar puncture sets. I imagine an ultrasound machine and the skilled hand to guide the probe over the abdomen to find the source of all the pain. I should be able to order a CT scanner or MRI. But I realize quickly that each of these things would be as misplaced here as an unplugged isolette stuffed with several small babies, an item that I do actually find in the nursery of the maternity hospital. JFK Hospital will need all of these things someday, before it can return to the sort of authority that it once had. But before that, and to make that possible, what I wish for them most fervently, for the doctors and medical students and their patients as well, is a library filled with books. They should have echocardiograms and infusion pumps, but first they should also have the sound of footsteps ringing on a smooth stone floor, the air cool and musty with the scent of ages that have gone past and the promise of a future that is to come. This was power, it was possibility, such knowledge only a finger's breadth away, and it was a library that I most longed to give them, knowing that from this all other things may grow.

Along the stretch of road between my hotel and the hospital gates, there are children walking home from school wearing matching blue skirts or trousers in combination with white tailored shirts. There is a boy, perhaps fifteen, pushing a wheelbarrow of small items that are for sale: a single roll of toilet paper, a neat metal disk containing shoeblack, and other soft clear plastic wrappers around fist-sized packages of nuts. I pass him each morning and a few short yards later I am greeted by a man and teenage boy sitting in a makeshift store, the shelves of the small shack stocked with cookies and other sugary snacks.

"Hello," they say and smile when I return the acknowledgment. "Hello." And I ask, "How are you?"

They answer, "Fine."

I have the same exchange, word for word, day after day, and week after week, with three girls around the age of five. At the roadside they sit putting red sandy earth into half of a bucket and pouring it out again. Their white teeth split their faces into wide and unembarrassed grins. The old woman sitting on a low rock some feet from them, her hair bound up in a piece of faded cloth, her thin legs folded into her caving chest, also says, "Hello."

It is only the white faces in this crowd of strangers who pointedly turn away, look straight ahead the way you might be taught to walk down the streets of New York or Geneva or Beruit, where blending in is possible, where anonymity might be both a blessing and a curse. A man runs by, his legs pale even with the tan, and he does not look at me. He does not ask after my health. I think that this must be how people do it, we passers-through, after they have been outsiders for so long. They refuse to see the alien passing beside them in order to not feel so alien themselves.

It is a silence I should perhaps have hid behind myself from the very start, a darkness around the eyes and a hard set to my lips that would have precluded others from making contact of any kind. It certainly would have been simpler. But then there would have been moments that I missed. If I had not smiled daily when I passed the phalanx of kindergarteners in their precious white and blue school uniforms, I would not have had the pleasure one morning of slapping all six of their extended right hands each in turn.

On the afternoon of my second day, I am determined to see the beach. The sea is visible, at no great distance, from the horizontally slotted windows of the pediatrics ward. I return to the hotel to deposit my laptop, change into a tank top, and smear some suntan lotion onto my face. I can see the ocean clearly through an opening in the wall at the end of my street, and I walk toward this, skirting the still expanse of sewage water green with algae that encircles the only manhole cover that I have seen. As I approach the opening in the concrete wall I had been headed for, I realize that it is blocked by the charred husk of an abandoned car. But now I see that there is another, smaller opening to the right on the other side of which

I would face a drop of more than a foot down onto the sand. It is a jump I might easily have taken, but I am stopped at first by the plentitude of garbage collected against the wall and on the beach just on the other side. Then I see the girl. She is laughing. What I see first is the side of her face, turning toward a friend; then I see her bare bottom as she squats to urinate. I move to one side, where she will not see me if she should turn back, for I do not want to cause embarrassment, and I wait. I consider whether I can safely negotiate the flattened cans and twists of wire and finally decide that I cannot, not without risking a cut that could easily become infected. I turn, and this time I see the first girl's companion, who is also taking a break to pee.

When I finally do reach the beach, several blocks in the direction of the hospital, there is even more garbage there. Two teenage boys are leaning against a dark blue pickup truck that has been driven out onto the place where small patches of grass give way to deeper sand. They stare as I go past. It is possible that they are there to fill the truck with refuse and to move it to another place, but if this is the case, then they are making no move to begin. When I pass later on my way back to the hotel, the truck is still standing where it had been parked, empty, and the boys are nowhere to be seen.

I carefully choose a place to sit, making sure that I see no glass or other sharp edges poking up between the coarse yellow and brown grains of sand. I also avoid the larger of the round holes that mark the entrances to the crab dens, small dark openings hidden on the edges of tiny hillocks and in the shadows cast by the mounds of sand, holes that are only an inch or so across and lead to the damp sanctuaries below. I fold a bright floral printed sarong and sit down, cross legged, on the square of fabric. In front of me the beach drops at a precipitous forty-five-degree angle along the irregular border that marks high tide, below which the sand has been washed back and forth so many times that it has been slowly carried away. The movement of the waves, as well, suggests that the drop might very well continue unseen, there beneath the wash of brown salt and foam, making this a dangerous place to swim. Elsewhere such a place might have been guarded by line drawings with the caption RIPTIDE in block letters just below. I realize then that the swimsuit I had packed does not belong here and I turn my head slightly to take in the scene again. Close to where I sit, an empty bag of saline still connected to IV tubing is half buried in the sand. Plastic bottles, only their noses visible, lie where they were cast weeks or years before. The beach is not some paradise to be photographed and stamped on postcards bordered in fluorescent pink. It is simply where the usable land ends and ocean beyond begins.

Behind me the houses bordering the beach are crumbling, and it is not just evidence of the passing of the years. The structures are made of cinder block or brick. They are missing walls, their windows are empty of screen or glass, and they are blackened in places as if a fire had swept through. They must have suffered some of this abuse during the war, when the men gathered and carried torches through the streets. A country with only a modest population, the city had filled to overflowing when the fighting began in earnest. They left their farms behind, fleeing the soldiers, and had moved here from the countryside to stay with relatives or to squat in the abandoned homes of those families with resources enough to move away. Monrovia may not have been safer than the rural areas, but it had felt that way.

"Even if you had a generator, you did not use it," Dr. Nuta says of those times. "You lit candles and you looked out of the windows at where other candles were lit. To use electricity, to actually turn on lights, would have been an advertisement that you had money, that you had things worth stealing. If you turned on lights and men came, they would not believe you if you told them the generator was all you had."

In the city, at least, there was no way to ever be alone, and the sounds of suffering that came from all around—the children crying, old women coughing, the men swearing at their wives—became in some strange way a source of comfort rather than distress.

It is beautiful, but not in the way that the well-groomed beaches of resorts manage to be, with their rows of pristine white lounge chairs and stretches of gentle and shallow turquoise surf. The place I stand is wild still, with the narrow ribbon of sand plunging too fast down toward the waves, which makes walking awkward, although not impossible. The water surges rapidly up the slope and the foam just as quickly recedes, causing small puffs of upward spray, like scores of tiny blowholes, to mark the turbulent flow over each of the openings where crabs are hiding within. When the water remains, for a time, safely below them, the holes are left behind as the incredibly camouflaged creatures emerge to scuttle about, defending their territory or in search of each diminutive morsel that has been whipped up onto their land. Glancing down, it is possible to believe that the sideways movements are only an illusion, a trick of the eye. Observed from farther off, the complicated dance gives the impression that it might have been generated on a computer by the same animators who depicted the Clone Armies in the latest *Star Wars*, with each iteration of the six-legged creatures an exact replica of the last.

I am sitting high on the sand with my legs hanging down the embankment when I meet Solomon. I close my book and look out at the water, intending to sit for only a short while before heading in. It is a mistake, this pause between lowering the shield of the open pages before me and standing to go, and he is there almost in the same moment that my defenses go down. He says hello and then sits down beside me.

"I have seen you before," he tells me and holds out his mobile phone. "This is you walking the other day, this is you sitting, and this is one I just took of you reading, and one looking."

There are perhaps half a dozen photos that flash each in succession onto the tiny screen. It is more than a little disquieting, but I sense that he has not meant this to make me uncomfortable, but as a form of flattery. It is even possible that he is just trying to show me that he has a nice phone. He tells me his name and that he works for the UN.

"You are not from Liberia?" I ask him.

"No. I am from Nigeria. I have been here three months. I came in March and I will be here until October 12, when my mission ends. I am proud to be here representing my country in this foreign mission for the UN."

The conversation is largely one-sided. I ask questions, having decided that this encounter, out in the open and as safe as is possible, is one of those things that travelers should embrace. Solomon answers. He tells me the number of his brothers and sisters but does not inquire if I have any of my own. He outlines how he had gone to university for a time and, lacking the money for fees, dropped out to join the Nigerian army. He does not ask my profession or what has brought me to Monrovia from wherever it is I've come. So I am surprised, given his lack of interest in my own life, at the way that he describes his love for his job, how it is an opportunity to meet so many people from all over the world. The truth is I am more than a little bored, for which I feel vaguely guilty. I make an excuse and move to go. The only thing he asks me directly is if I am married and I tell him that I am. I rub absently at the place where for two years my diamond wedding band had rested but that I had removed before coming, judging it an ironic but unnecessary risk to bring these gems into the same country from which they might have come.

Solomon is there waiting the next time I come to the beach. Before I quite know what has happened, his arms are around me in a full-bodied embrace and then he has stepped back and is holding both my hands in his own. Several days have gone past since our last meeting, a stilted exchange that lasted on the whole perhaps fifteen minutes, and he remarks on my absence as if it needs to be explained.

I reclaim my hands on the pretext of having to adjust the strap of my bag across my shoulder and then jam them deep into my pockets. I should appreciate his friendliness, his hospitality to another traveler who is far from home, but instead I feel distinctly uncomfortable, realizing all at once just how vulnerable I have become.

He waves to his friends with a wide smile, revealing the gap between both his upper and lower two front teeth, the result perhaps of sucking on too much sugarcane. Then he introduces me to the other soldiers, young men in uniform who are from Ghana and Bangladesh. In the process of asking for my phone number, he wonders aloud if my husband realizes how lucky he is to be married to a white woman and I decide that I am done. The color of my skin is not, as far as I am aware, anywhere on the list of reasons my husband decided it would make him happy to spend our lives together. I lie and tell Solomon that I do not have a phone. He is disappointed but insists on finding a small scrap of paper upon which to write his own numbers, the one he is using while he is in Liberia, and his Nigerian number for when I call him after October, after he has gone home. His eyes wide and childlike, it is as if he is willing me to fall into the illusion he has created, that we might be friends, that he might actually be someone I would choose to call.

"They want green cards," Dr. Dennis says casually one day. "That's why they're so excited to meet Americans. They believe you have the power to help them."

It is all too clear to me how far short I fall from this expectation. I don't even have the power to help the children who arrive at the hospital, walking barefoot in the dust beside their grandmothers or tied tight with cloth over the old woman's back. Whatever illusions I had nurtured that I would find some higher calling here have been dissipated quickly. It does no good to know the right dose of a medication that a child should be getting for his asthma flare if there is not a pharmacy in the whole country that can provide it. Neither can I help the starving toddler with the swollen belly by my knowing what protein and vitamin deficiencies he clearly suffers from, when I have no way of providing a reliable source of that nutrition. So though I am more than simply the white woman who Solomon takes me for, I am less than that, as well. Standing before Solomon as he holds out his phone number, I do not know how to be honest. I do not know how to be friends because I do not know how to make him see me for who I really am. I know that I will not call him, but with the eyes of his fellow soldiers upon us, I take the paper he hands me and walk away.

Later that week, it rains during my morning walk to the hospital.

"I can have one of the drivers come pick you up tomorrow morning," Dr. Dennis tells me on the afternoon of my first day.

I defer, ostensibly to avoid being a burden but also because I want the luxury of setting my own schedule in the mornings and the time alone during my walk.

"Make sure you call if it is raining. You shouldn't walk in all that wet."

But I don't call. I look out at the pavement, already wet from the night's onslaught, and up at the clouded but bright sky. It is only a weak spatter of a shower that is coming down, so I press the button to release the catch on my umbrella and lift its periwinkle dome above me. I have gone perhaps two blocks when the pattering on the light blue nylon shield becomes more insistent. I keep walking forward briskly, head down with my free arm cradling my laptop case before me, attempting to keep it somewhat drier than my backside increasingly is becoming. Then, seemingly without warning (although this is certainly what Dr. Dennis had meant when he reminded me this was the rainy season), the rain comes down in sheets. It is a roar as insistent and as constant as the blood behind your ears after heavy exertion, and as if to acknowledge this, I can taste iron on the back of my tongue.

In less than a minute, my skirt is sodden from the knees down and my black flats are filled with water that squelches between my toes. Cars move past me slowly, as if mired in the effort to displace the liquid before them or like a swimmer carrying a heavy stone as he walks across the bottom of a pool. The noise is deafening. I do not hear the crunch of tires on the wet gravel or the splash as cars roll through puddles that are becoming ever wider and even more deep. I barely even hear the horn, although the car is right beside me. Then it stops. I know that I can neither make it to the hospital nor back to the hotel without risking serious damage to my computer. I duck and open the car door. Once seated, I see the JFK Hospital sticker on the windshield and recognize the uniform of one of the hospital drivers, but the truth is I hadn't seen the sticker through the rain. I did not know the man by sight and I didn't care. I would have gotten into a car with anyone.

I am still drying off when I see a child in the clinic who had been prophetically named Handful after she was born. The girl's mother is dead. Across the desk from me, her grandmother (afraid enough to bring the child to the hospital but not yet ready to hear the words spoken aloud) grasps the one-year-old to her, the child no bigger than she should have been three or four months earlier. The grandmother says that maybe the girl is skinny because she does not get the right foods, because she eats mostly a paste made from cassava that is called *fufu*. Maybe it is her own fault for not having the right things to feed her, to fatten her up. Even at first glance, the child's skin is dry but at the same time bears a worrisome oily sheen. Then the grandmother removes the diaper, a cloth tucked through the infant's legs and tied in place with a thin plastic sheet. I lean closer to look at the horrible rash that had been hidden beneath.

"How did her mother die?" I ask, not because I am cruel, but because it is important.

The child's grandmother lifts her shoulders with a suggestion of bewilderment.

"She got sick. For three months she was sick and then she died."

"What was it?" I ask again.

"Malaria," she tells me, and I know that Handful needs to be tested for HIV.

I tell her grandmother that it is always safest, really, to rule out the bigger things that could be wrong. This is true. Then I tell her that if the tests come back positive and Handful does have HIV, the hospital will make sure she gets the medicines she will need.

This is an awful moment, because I know that no matter what medicines she is given, Handful will surely die. Both at Children's and at the City Hospital, doctors struggle with how to take care of teenagers who have HIV. There are not many of them, but there are some who contracted the virus from their mothers before they were born. Now these children must return home from school on time each day so that they can swallow their pills. The crisis, the hot topic, is how to transition these teenagers into adulthood, how to guide them with sensitivity into being ready for intimate relationships, all the while instilling within them the responsibility to use condoms, because sex with them can kill. Handful will not get to be one of those teens, angry at the world and experimenting with drugs. Instead, she will waste away to practically nothing and one day get a fever, and another day she will be gone.

But her grandmother is here and that is something. Earlier that same day, there had been a mother with her newborn, a three-day-old with a fever of 102. I usually think of my job as reassuring parents while trying to teach them, but for this mother, determined to leave the clinic with the child and blindly refusing admission, I pull out all the stops. "I know it is hard to be here, and we would send you home if we thought that it was safe. But I really believe that the baby will get worse and not better, and he could die before you can bring him back. The infection could go to his brain or to his blood and that can kill him."

"He could die," I say again because she is not hearing the words, is looking at me with defiance and none of the trust to which I am accustomed. Then she takes the baby away.

As with this earlier patient, Handful's grandmother and I have only a few minutes to sit across from each other and talk. I can offer her no more good news than I did that mother with her infant daughter. Still she is meeting my gaze eagerly, and though her back is repeatedly brushed against in this narrow space by people trying to get by, she does not look away. I do not have any real idea what she understands of what I have told her, but she repeats back to me the time and the place she is to bring Handful for the blood testing and for the follow-up appointment with the infectious disease staff. Then she gathers up the small bundle that is her only granddaughter and she carries Handful home.

Leaving the hospital on that day, I feel the defeat pound at me like the small fishing boats visible from the beach are pounded by the waves.

Besides Handful, there had also been the one-year-old who will never walk. He was born with two club feet and oddly angled legs and hips that are dislocated on both sides. His hands are also turned in as if he grew inside his mother's belly with not enough room to move. It is possible that this is what has happened. His mother had no prenatal care and never had an ultrasound to measure how much fluid she had inside. If this is the reason the child's limbs are improperly formed, then he may have kidney or lung problems as well. They are problems we can do nothing for in this place, so I tell his mother that she should give him plenty of good food to keep his lungs as healthy as she can. Even if his lungs are healthy, there are some problems it is just not possible to fix.

At Children's, his parents would have asked if their child would ever walk. They would have been offered painful surgeries and his bones would have been broken in a multitude of places and then pieced back together again. Maybe then he would have been able to bear his weight, but it would not have been an achievement purchased for free. It would have hurt, the surgery itself and the long physical therapy after, and in some ways (the boy sitting comfortably on his deformed legs in a chair before me) I am not sorry that this sort of aggressive treatment is not one I can give. He has family to move him from one place to another. And though the way in which he crawls forward dragging his legs behind him is certainly awkward, it does not seem to cause him pain.

And there was the boy with the tumor on the right side of his face, stretching the skin and bubbling outward as if at any moment it might burst through. For these three, the antimalarials and deworming medicines I have at my disposal will not do any good. I try in vain to swallow my frustration and to imagine how I would feel if this place were my home.

On one of my first afternoons, I asked Trokon what he wanted to do after medical school. We talked for more than an hour, sitting in the dark when the electricity went out and the generator failed to turn on, his face and eyes hidden in the shadows, the only indication of his position the occasional flash of white when his lips broke into a smile. It had been more than ten years since he graduated high school and entered university, but his studies were interrupted many times because of the war. When the fighting was too close, or when the professors given the responsibility for teaching certain courses left the country in search of safety and more reliable salaries, the medical students had remained in the dormitories, poring over tattered, dog-eared books left behind by visitors, their lives essentially on hold.

"Will you stay here after your internship?" I asked him.

When Trokon answered, it was the shrug that said it all, the dim outline of his shoulders illuminated by a faint sliver of light crawling beneath the door. He did not say that he wanted to go, but neither did he promise that he will stay.

"You have seen what it is like here. Soon I will be thirty. I need to make money."

And, on another day, "When we say *family*, it is not the way you mean it. I have been supported by my family for all these years. It is not just my parents, who have nine children. It is my uncles and aunts. When I do graduate, they will look at me and say, 'Now you are a doctor. Now you can take care of us.' It is not enough, what they pay us here, to do this. So people have gone to England or South Africa or Australia. Many dream of going to the United States. Then you can send money back. I think some will stay, but many will choose to go because they have to."

Dr. Dennis, on the other hand, looks at the problem very differently. He can tell me at any given moment exactly how many native doctors are within his country's borders, how many foreigners, how many of them are actually practicing medicine as opposed to performing administrative duties or doing projects in public health. It is a number that is far from equal to the task of providing basic services to the population.

"Our only urologist is in his seventies. Our only ENT is blind," he says. "My wife is still an anesthesiologist in DC, so she can pay our children's college tuition. So when they asked me to come back to run the hospital, how could I possibly have refused?"

In the dormitory at the medical school, the electricity has gone out because no one has paid the bill. They still have water, Trokon claims, because President Johnson Sirleaf gave them the water as a gift. She came to the medical school campus and met them. There are 120 doctors in this country of 3.5 million. Only 75 or so are Liberians, and many are working for NGOs (nongovernmental organizations) and not seeing patients. There is no pediatrician in the whole of the country, only consultants who claim an expertise in pediatrics by virtue of having practiced on children for so many years.

It used to be that patients were sent to JFK Hospital from Ghana and Sierra Leone to see the specialists there. Now Dr. Dennis is trying to arrange for the residents to go to study in Ghana and then to bring that knowledge home. If the wealth of a nation is really her people, then certainly these few remaining medical students deserve at the very least a little electricity so that they can blow out their candles and turn on the lights.

Already Trokon's class is half the size it was when they began. There are thirteen who will graduate when another year has passed. When this year finishes, only four will move on to their internships from the class that is just one step ahead. It is the war, in part. It is the waiting for their lives to begin, a need to be unstuck in time that is just part of growing up. The ones who drop out leave because they wanted cars and jobs, not because they stopped loving medicine. But medicine is not what they had thought it would be when they started. People were dying, from the war and from starvation and from maladies they knew from books should be easy for them to fix. The ones who left were tired of gambling on a university and hospital that were not giving them the skills they knew they would need, and they had not wanted to be there in the middle of the night forced to stand helpless amid the screams.

One Saturday, Trokon brings me a basket of fruit. I had asked where I might buy some mangoes, and this was his response. I meet him at the administrative building and he shyly opens the top of the blue plastic basket to reveal the plunder inside. There are ripe mangoes, oranges, pears, and bananas. It is more fruit than any one person can eat, but I thank him profusely, because such generosity is overwhelming in this place where people count themselves lucky if they are able to eat two times a day. After we have examined in full the contents of the container, he opens a black plastic bag and pulls back the edges to reveal the top of an enormous pineapple.

"It is getting spoiled in the heat," he says with frank disappointment.

I reassure Trokon that it is a wonderful gift and that I will carry it back to where I am staying and put it someplace cool. Back in my hotel, I drop the pineapple into my bathroom sink and cut it in half by making deep jabbing motions with a butter knife. I hack out pieces of the sweet fruit and slice away the rot. It tastes even better because of the ridiculous struggle with which I cut it. By the time I have completed the task, the bathroom floor is wet from the sugary spray and my feet adhere noisily to the tile. Next I eat a mango, pulling the strings of pulp away from the long ellipse of the stone. I shower when I have finished, having managed to become tacky practically from head to foot, and wash the sticky sweetness away.

We have our first sickler the second week I am there. I am surprised actually that it has taken this long. The girl, Wonlay, appears on the ward one morning during rounds. She is fourteen and she would be gangly if she could hold herself upright. Her long legs hang over the edges of the crib and she moans and twists herself upon the thin stained sheet. One leg is significantly swollen just above the knee. She clutches it as she turns again, supporting the leg and then placing it down, struggling to find a position that does not cause her whole limb to burn. Her tissues are dying. Some balance has been lost. Whether through dehydration or bad luck, a few red blood cells had started to sickle, the crescent moon-shaped cells becoming lodged within the smaller venules, creating ischemia and prompting the sickling of other cells in turn. When this happens in the lungs, the patient cannot breathe, which is the most common cause of death for these children. For Wonlay, it is only her leg, and it is unlikely to kill her, but I doubt this is something that she would find comforting during the red hot flashes of pain.

At the City Hospital and even at Children's, there are nearly always a small handful of children in vaso-occlusive pain crisis, the fragile sickled red cells lacking the flexibility to make it through the smaller vessels at the tips of their fingers or deep inside their bones. In the ER, these children are given generous doses of IV morphine or Dilaudid, the same doses that would snow a larger man, barely breaking through their pain. They are hooked up to PCA machines as quickly as possible, with a slow continuous infusion and a button to press for when that basal rate is not enough. We treat the sicklers quickly because we know they will have the pain again, because they have enough obstacles to success in the missed days of school and the accumulation of small, imperceptible strokes that are working away at the insides of their brains. They should not have to live every moment in between in fear of how bad the pain will be the next time it returns.

Interestingly, Wonlay's moaning has in some perverse way lightened the mood on the ward. The silence that had been so characteristic of these morning rounds has been shattered. It is as if Wonlay's involuntary utterances, rising as they do at times almost to a scream, have given to those around her a freedom while signaling the prison she is in. Mothers are talking and passing each other bowls of food between the cribs. Two children admitted for malaria but obviously ready to go home take turns slapping each other lightly on the arm and then running away.

I have learned to phrase my questions without judgment, although I feel as surely in my own flesh as Wonlay feels the pain in hers that it is a crime just to watch her lying there.

"Do you ever give opiates to these patients?"

She is getting only paracetamol and some IV fluids to dilute her blood.

Dr. Andrews shakes her head.

"We don't ever do that," but she does not offer an explanation why.

After rounds, in Dr. Dennis's office, I tell him about Wonlay. I had made sure that she was getting ibuprofen at least, for its anti-inflammatory effects, even while knowing how far this is from actually being enough.

"The pharmacy doesn't have any morphine," he admits. "The real shame is that you can buy morphine from those guys who push the wheelbarrows. We call them wheelbarrow pharmacies."

"So she would be getting better pain control at home," I say, and it is not a question.

Dr. Dennis does not contradict me.

"What are the women getting after their C-sections?" I ask, afraid that I already know the answer.

He releases a low, grim chuckle. "Paracetamol," naming a drug that is no different from Tylenol.

"I am never, ever, having a baby here."

He laughs, with a real smile this time. "I know a doctor who calls this the house of pain. I don't think that's fair."

Life isn't fair, I think looking around me, but I do not say.

In the nursery there is a baby who is dying. On the warmer next to her is an infant who is already dead. I was not present for this death; I arrive a few minutes after the gasping has finished, and her heart, starved of oxygen, finally stops. On the peds ward, I had been giving a lecture on pediatric GU (genitourinary) emergencies. There had been pictures. I had said the word penis far too many times to be comfortable, but I had struggled through it while Dr. Nuta's cell phone rang, and she, without any apparent sense of urgency, had ducked out of the room. I wonder if she had dawdled. It is possible that along the pavement between the side entrance to the main hospital and the maternity building across the way, or while walking the back path lined with coils of razor wire (sheets laid carefully over their sharp edges to dry in the sun), she had stopped for a while. I imagine it would have been tempting to do this, knowing that whatever she found in the NICU when she arrived, there would be nothing she was able to do.

The baby had been breathing fast shallow breaths sucked in through his open mouth. What he needed was CPAP, applied gently with an anesthesia bag and a mask. What he needed was to be intubated and to have surfactant poured down the tube to lubricate his immature lungs. He needed these things, but he would never receive them here; the resources were just not available. By the time he began sharply sucking in the hollow of his neck and the spaces in between each of his ribs, it was already too late. It was too late when his mother's labor began and the bag he was swimming in broke wide open in a warm rush to deliver him too soon. This would, in no small way, be torture to witness. So I would not have blamed Dr. Nuta if her feet dragged.

At home at least, I would have immediately sprinted down the hall, secure in the knowledge that there was work to be done. I would have run and burst through the door, and there would have been the warmer and oxygen supply and bulb suction, the bag mask and laryngoscope and ET tube, waiting for me. There would have been in that room the possibility of action, of rescue, and I would have run lest I arrive too late. But there is nothing like this kind of promise waiting in the room to which Dr. Nuta had headed, where I meet her just after, and where I take hold of one limp, not yet cold, perfect foot. I pass my thumb over the wrinkles of the sole and count all five blessed half-moons of each tiny nail. He is hardly the first child who has died since my arrival, but he is the first I have actually touched.

The first child, the HIV-positive toddler (though he never had enough strength to learn how to toddle), had simply disappeared in the space of the night. So, too, the newborn with bilateral clefts in his lip and his soft palate, dead only hours after his mother first agreed to finally hold him. And there were the children who came into the ER and died in that horrible pungent collection of connected rooms on the ground floor. They died of AIDs or of dehydration; they died of perforations in their bowel caused by typhoid or from malaria parasites that had traveled insidiously to infect their brains. In some ways these deaths were a relief in their quickness. By the time most of these children were brought in for care, they were poised on the precipice and there was no way in the end to stop their fall. The lingering had been done elsewhere, so it was possible to pretend that their deaths were inevitable, that no one was at fault.

It is much more difficult to watch the infant named Wollie remain unconscious for the entire month that I am there. I meet her in the first few days after my arrival. She is at that time about six hours old and on oxygen. Dr. Nuta and Dr. Andrews are looking through the stapled papers, noting her Apgars, the time she was first noted to have respiratory distress. They would have seen many such infants the nights they took call alone in the hospital during their yearlong internship. But unlike the nights I spent trailing behind my senior resident, they had had no one to learn from, so they remain unsure about much of what they do. They look up at me. There is a silence while I wait first to see if either one of them wishes to say something.

When it seems that they don't, I say, "She needs antibiotics. I would start amp and gent."

She spikes her first fever later that night and continues to be febrile, despite antibiotics, for at least two weeks more. On the third day, I realize that she was not actually being fed; the only thing she was receiving was the liquid infusion of her antibiotics. I quickly write for a bolus and daily IV fluids and wonder what else we'd all missed. During this first seventy-two hours, she does not pass urine and her bladder distension only worsens, so I press a needle into her abdomen just above the pubic bone. I draw back on the plastic syringe I am holding, but no urine comes out. I leave the nurse to hang the fluids. Several hours later an intern pokes another needle, perhaps an inch below the drying stump of the infant's umbilical cord, not the safest place and not where the textbooks instruct to, but by this time the bladder is so bloated that it is pressed up against the inside of the abdominal wall and no bowel intervenes. Several days after this second suprapubic tap, she begins urinating on her own. Surprisingly, her fever becomes only intermittent and she is breathing comfortably on room air. The crisis seems to have passed by the time she is a week old, but she remains limp and unresponsive. She moves her arms and legs only in response to pain, and then only slightly, as if the pain has only just barely reached that part of her brain that continues to rally on.

Wollie lies on one of three radiant warmers, their electric coils turned off and in all likelihood broken, but beds that are stifling nonetheless in the blistering heat of the windowless room. While Wollie continues to receive antibiotics and fluids dripped into her vein, the warmers beside her are home to a succession of small squirming newborns. They are given oxygen as they struggle to take in enough air despite lungs still heavy with fluid, the alveoli too immature to expand without enormous resistance, so with each painful breath, the pitiful curve of their ribs stands out in stark relief. Wollie breathes comfortably, but remains disturbingly still. While these newcomers struggle, the solitary nurse in charge of these infants stands watch or (more often) sits just outside the door to catch some of the breeze that comes in from the sea.

On occasion, Wollie's mother holds her and puts her to the breast. For several days she has been fed breast milk through an NG tube, milk that was kneaded down toward the nipple and squeezed out drop by drop. When Wollie is two weeks old, I first hear the murmur when I place my stethoscope on her small chest. I am fairly certain that it was not there before. It is possible that whatever microbe is the source of her infection has made its way to the valves of her heart, causing damage there, so blood sloshes back and forth as the muscle contracts. She is afebrile, but I continue the antibiotics through the weekend; at the start of my last week, I tell the nurse to finally stop. Off all medications, we watch her for any recurrence of the high temperature, but she remains just as she is, not awake or asleep, unmoving except in response to a finger pressed firmly against her palm. This prompts her only to weakly curl her fingers but not to hold on.

In my third week I open up my laptop to give a lecture on antibiotic resistance and soft-tissue infections. Even if there is not now a high prevalence of antibiotic-resistant bacteria lurking silently in the moist armpits or groins of men and women in this country where you can buy antibiotics on the street corners—selecting amoxicillin or metronidazole from among the toilet paper rolls and toothpaste piled into these wheelbarrows—there surely soon will be. I am on a soapbox, but it is a disaster (nothing less) that I know is coming, worse than the disaster that is already here. Most families struggle to afford Bactrim, amoxicillin, and ceftriaxone. They will surely not be able to afford vancomycin and linezolid once resistant strains of bacteria become commonplace.

Robert, another one of the medical students, interrupts my lecture to tell me that a new patient has arrived. He had been sent up from the ER without warning, which is simply the way things work. At Children's, there would have been pages and multiple phone calls. The attendings would have signed out to each other, the residents as well, and the nurses in the ER would have let those waiting on the floor know exactly what the patient needed, exactly when the elevator doors slid shut. It would have been clear, at any given moment, just whose responsibility the child was. This infant who has just arrived exists in a sort of gray zone, a shadowy realm of light and darkness, where nothing really is real, no one really in charge. Except the child is real, despite our knowing nothing about him, and he is clearly far from well.

Robert is apologetic as he catches my attention. On my laptop screen there is a picture of a petri dish with antibiotic-laden disks dropped on a lawn of *Staph aureus* and the circles that show which drugs still work. I stand and walk out of the nurses' room into the main bay of the ward, the students trailing along behind me, one of them taking the time to carefully hide my computer in a drawer from which it will not be taken by any passersby. There are student nurses clustered around the crib, making jabbing motions toward the child, who is still hidden from my view. One thrusts a thermometer beneath his armpit; one viciously swipes a cool damp cloth across his sweaty brow. He is six months old, and in the ER he had been diagnosed with malaria. The fluorescent pee-colored quinine infusion is already hanging and running into a vein on the right side of his scalp.

I have to speak loudly in order to reach the boy, weaving my arms between the nurses until eventually my body is allowed to follow. The boy is breathing fast, is sucking desperately at the air, as I place the stethoscope on his chest to listen, and in his struggle to breathe I mistake his distress for asthma without any history of what happened downstairs.

When I step back, the opening I had made is quickly closed again. I write some orders for breathing medicines in his chart and hand them to a nurse.

"We need to get these medications from the pharmacy right away," I say urgently.

She tells me that his hemoglobin is low, that they ordered a transfusion when they evaluated him downstairs.

"That's not what's important right now. He'll get the blood, but I need you to get these medications from the pharmacy right now."

Behind the wall of people between me and the child, someone says, "He's convulsing."

I push one of the nursing students out of my way, write for diazepam, and send another nurse to get it. The child's eyes roll back in his head and his body twitches but does not jerk as violently as I know it might. His breathing is still labored, is getting worse, and instead of simply breathing quickly, he pauses for five seconds at a time and then starts to pant again. I realize then that the coarse breath sounds I had heard when I first listened were the result of saliva that had been sucked into his lungs when he was seizing.

"We need to get an oxygen sat," I say loudly to cut over the noise of other voices.

"The respiratory therapists will need to be called," Trokon says.

I shake my head without looking at him.

"There's a machine in the cardiac patient's crib," I say, referring to a small boy in the last room with a congenital heart defect who has been living in the hospital for months while being given oxygen despite the fact that his heart will in all likelihood never be fixed. I had seen the sat machine there less than an hour before. Trokon leaves to get it while one of the nurses inexplicably pours cold water over the new patient until he is lying in a puddle on the plastic mattress of the crib. The nurse I sent for diazepam returns, and by the time Trokon appears with the sat machine, the diazepam is being given through the scalp IV. But there is no electrical outlet close enough to reach this crib. As the pauses in the boy's breathing become more frightening, now that he has received the sedating IV diazepam and the seizure has been stopped, we move him to another crib, one closer to an outlet so that we can plug things in. The sat machine is turned on and the probe placed on his toe. It reads somewhere in the mid-80s. His heart rate is 210. He is sucking harder to take each breath and I reach down to shove a wad of fabric beneath his shoulders to accentuate the backward tilt of his head.

I listen to his chest again and then try to summarize: "His sats are low and he needs oxygen."

"The respiratory therapists are looking for a mixer," one of the medical students interjects.

"Okay," I say, my left hand pressing down on his forehead and my right lifting his jaw to keep his airway wide open. "For now he's breathing on his own, but he's having brief apneic spells and he's not moving very good air. This is probably because he aspirated when he was seizing and also because the diazepam we gave can suppress the respiratory drive. His heart rate is high, but he's young, and as long as he has a healthy heart, then this is sustainable for at least a little while. It's likely high because of the stress of the seizure and his respiratory distress and also because he's very anemic, which is why he will be getting blood."

I hear the steady chirping of the sat machine drop minutely in its pitch. From where I am standing, I cannot see the screen.

"Robert, you're going to keep telling what his sats are."

"It's 81," he tells me quickly.

The pauses in the infant's breathing are becoming longer. When I listen, only one breath in five is moving air. I flick the bottom of his sole hard to encourage the intake of air.

"Do we have a bag and mask?"

"The respiratory therapist is getting oxygen," I am told, which is not at all what I just asked.

"Is there a bag and mask anywhere on the ward?" I ask again, still attacking the pale sole of the infant's foot, hoping to stimulate him.

"No. There might be one in the respiratory therapists' office."

"Then you need to go and get it." Smith leaves the bedside and I again ask Robert to tell me the boy's sat. It is stable in the 80s, but falls whenever I stop flicking the child's foot. One of the respiratory therapists comes by to say that the oxygen machine he went to get was being used and it might take a while to get one from the nursery.

I stop for a moment my attack on the poor infant's sole to look the respiratory therapist in the eye and say, "This baby could die in the next few minutes. He needs oxygen as quickly as you can get it."

I do not watch him leave the room but look down again at the rise and fall of the small chest below me. He breathes for ten seconds at a time and then stops for five and then breathes for ten seconds more. It is not enough and the pitch of the sat machine's beeping is falling steadily.

"Who do you call when you need help?" I ask, but no one answers. It is not because they haven't heard; it is because they do not know, because there is no one else to call.

At Children's, it is standing room only, each code a highly attended event. The ICU team takes charge as soon as they arrive; the anesthesiologists secure the airway if it is a particularly tricky case. In the last two years, I had been the first to arrive at only one such affair and I had called for help almost the moment I walked into the room.

"His sat," I prompt Robert.

Robert says, "80, . . . 75."

My eyes settle on the round O of the infant's mouth, the flaring nostrils, the dusky lips. I squeeze his nose shut between my left thumb and index finger.

"Seventy," Robert tells me.

I put my mouth over this infant whose name I do not know and I breathe out, slowly, then pull back and then breathe out again. I straighten for a moment and Smith reappears, a self-inflating bag and mask in his hand. I tell Trokon how to hold the head for me and I press the mask onto his face, covering his mouth and nose. I squeeze the bag, too quickly, I know, giving him a breath every two seconds instead of every four, until his sats begin to respond.

He comes up to the 90s, and I look at Smith: "Do you want to bag?"

He nods, "Yes," and takes it from me.

"I want your fingers in a C shape so you can press down and keep the air from leaking out. That's good."

We bag the infant until the oxygen comes and then uncoil the tubing from the bag mask assembly to hook it up to oxygen flow.

"Smith, I want you to give him only one breath every four seconds now that we have oxygen and we'll see how he does."

Smith squeezes the bag more slowly, the bare chest rises and it falls, not always in harmony with the breaths that we are giving, but for now it is enough. When thirty seconds or so have passed, I tell

Smith to hold the breaths but to leave the oxygen mask close up to the infant's face. The sats remain stable in the 90s and we unplug the bag mask from the oxygen supply.

"Take the mask off his face," I tell Smith, "or he'll suffocate, now that the oxygen is not connected."

Smith withdraws his hand while the respiratory therapist attaches a face mask to the oxygen mixer and slips the mask's elastic cord behind the boy's small head. He is still breathing irregularly and his lung sounds are coarse and diminished throughout, but with the help of the oxygen he is holding his own.

I mistake the woman with eyes red from crying for his mother, not guessing that she might be his grandmother because she looks so young. I gesture to her to come to the bedside, now that the crowd has thinned.

"You can touch him," I tell her, and she reaches out to take his hand.

"He's not awake," I tell her.

And she says, "No," as if I have asked a question.

"In Africa," his aunt will tell me a few hours later, "when we see oxygen on a child, we think that he must die. Is that always true?"

I try to make my voice as gentle as I can when I tell her, "No. We wouldn't give the oxygen if we didn't think that it would help. I think his lungs are damaged and I think that they will get better slowly, but I do think they'll get better. The oxygen is just to make sure that even while his lungs aren't working properly, he's getting enough oxygen into his blood."

"Thank you," she says, and I place one hand on her shoulder in encouragement.

But on the second night of his hospitalization, after having improved greatly, he has another seizure or cluster of seizures lasting several hours. The following morning, his lungs sound horrendous, with the coarse fluttering of mucus audible as he moves air in and out. And whereas he had demonstrated some minimal level of awareness the evening before, this morning following the prolonged seizure, he does not stir at all.

His mother and grandmother continue to take shifts by his bedside, wiping the saliva as it drips from the corners of his lips and dries on his chin and cheeks. Despite this, they continue to thank me every day after we have finished rounds until the day that I go home.

"Doc, can you do an exam?" Trokon asks me while he scribbles his note and gestures to the mother of the three-year-old boy that she should place him on the table. He has not yet examined the child, but is instead still scratching notes on what the boy's mother has told him on the single white piece of paper stapled into the boy's chart.

The medical students are too harried to muster any real interest in learning from what they are doing, pressed into this small cubicle without any regular supervision and expected to move quickly through each of the patients waiting on the long wooden benches that line the halls just outside. These mothers have walked hours with a small child tied onto their back and one or two others dawdling behind. They deserve more than a few minutes of a student's time for such effort, but it is all they will get, and even then the motions will be gone through much by rote. Any child with a fever will be prescribed medication for malaria. Ear infections, so common in the private pediatricians' offices at home, do not exist here, because there are no instruments to diagnose it. And viral infections, the cause of so many fevers, are not acknowledged or recognized. I have wondered repeatedly how to set a different tone to these clinic visits, how to encourage the students to examine carefully each of their patients before I do and then tell me what they think. But there is just no way to slow down the session and not risk leaving children still waiting, unseen, when the clinic is shut down when the electricity goes out.

I would like to tell Trokon to examine the boy himself, but there is no time to argue. I have been paying only partial attention to the conversation he has been having with the boy's mother, busy instead with another student's patient, an infant with a disturbingly swollen arm. This baby should be referred to the surgical clinic where the bone can be set and casted, but first he needs something for his pain. We have just finished up a lengthy discussion, the result of which was the revelation that there was really nothing available that he could be given without writing out a prescription and asking the mother to get the medication herself.

I help lift Trokon's patient onto the examination table, placing him straight down on the dirty sheet that has been spread over the slippery and torn vinyl covering beneath. I perform my exam and stop with my fingers pressed into the soft flesh just below the boy's navel. I turn and try to catch Trokon's eye without speaking because I do not want the child's mother to hear the alarm that I know would be in my voice.

Trokon does not look up, so I palpate the abdomen again, stepping my fingers over the edge of the mass, a smooth and hard barrier to my probing hands.

As casually as I can, I say, "I think you should come examine him."

Trokon extricates himself from behind the bulky desk, brushing up against yet another dirty sheet that has been inexplicably laid over a surface with too little friction to hold it in place. He feels the mass and asks what needs to be done.

He needs a CT scan, I think to myself, but say, "He needs an abdominal ultrasound. Will they do it today?"

Trokon looks unconvinced; there is a furrow of displeasure that appears at the center of his brow.

"It is late," he says, although it is not yet one o'clock in the afternoon.

"And if I went with them?" I suggest, reluctant to admit that this might matter but knowing that it does.

"They might do it," he agrees.

So we sit, the boy and his mother and I, on the long bench in the unlit corridor outside the radiologist's office. At first we are led into the office by the technician manning the waiting area. I proceed to introduce the child, explaining that he needs to see the surgeons as soon as possible but will need imaging of his abdomen before this can be done.

Dr. Oputa does not answer me but instead gestures to the man sitting across the desk from him: "I am talking with this gentleman here."

I apologize, profusely and out of proportion to the offense, hoping to garner enough good favor to get the ultrasound done. Outside of the office we sit and the minutes drain from us like sweat. After more than thirty minutes of waiting, Dr. Oputa emerges and looks around at the benches on either side of the corridor, finally settling on my white face.

"What were you saying?" he asks me, and I repeat the story I have already told.

He looks at his watch, which if it is keeping appropriate time, cannot tell him that it is much after two. "We usually close down around now, but you are a visitor and we don't want you to be disappointed."

I could slap him hard across the face and with enough force to draw blood from his teeth on the inside of his cheek, and I hate him for stepping so neatly into the cliché. I have less than a week remaining before I am due back at Children's, where this will be a test that I easily could get. Still, I notice that he has not actually agreed yet to do the study and I add, "I was hoping if you can do the ultrasound that you might let me watch. I've never been able to look at something like this before."

He nods slowly then, and a third chin appears beneath the other two. "This way."

With the probe pressed firmly against the child's abdomen, we can see his bladder, the hepatic and portal veins passing into his liver, the flash of the valves as they open and close within his beating heart. Then the probe is placed over the tumor. Dr. Oputa shakes his head and repositions his hand, twisting a dial on the monitor before him.

"These machines you send us from the West. They are more trouble than they are worth."

I nod agreeably, hoping that he will condescend to spend at least a few minutes more defining the edges of the mass, determining if it has infiltrated the renal vein. But he waves the probe in the air and declares, "It is broken. He should come back tomorrow. I will use a better machine."

The child's mother does come back, two or three more times, but it is always the same and eventually they give up. They never see the surgeon. His tumor will grow until it presses his liver up against his right lung. The mere volume of it will cut off all passage of stool. He will vomit. He will lose weight and become dehydrated. Then he will die. It is already too late by the time that I see him, by the time the first cancerous cell started to divide. I know this, but I can do nothing. I sometimes look for him, in those final days when I walk past a bench full of waiting parents and their children. I think of him often. It is hardly enough.

As I get ready to leave Liberia, I am not sure that I have become a better doctor. It is not clear to me, in fact, whether anything has really changed. I have stood powerless over too many dying children to think about this time except in the smallest of pieces, snapshots with blurry edges taken from too close up or else at a great distance through a distorting lens. Sitting in the airport before a television screen, I watch Nelson Mandela take the stage at his ninetieth birthday celebration. Will and Jada Pinkett Smith shout his name and then step aside. As the Hyde Park crowd cheers and raises their hands out toward him, I know that the things that most need changing—the bellies empty of sustenance and the minds empty of dreams—I have not even touched.

I feel reduced somehow, hardened, like a clay brick set out to bake in the sun. In the midst of the chaos, there had been at least one moment when my mind and my actions had been completely uncluttered. I fix on this memory as I walk across the tarmac and take my seat on the plane. With the seizure broken and the child lying breathless before me, the orchestrated drills, the CPR dummies, and the laminated yellow code cards were thousands of miles away. So I breathed out so that his lungs could fill. There was the risk of infection, but there was nothing else to do in that moment but press my lips over his. I breathed. And then so did he, for a while. I had not saved him, but during the past weeks I realized that this was not why I had come.

Liberia is in need of doctors, certainly, but doctors who will stay. Before I leave, I give a stethoscope to Trokon, knowing that his own rendered even the obvious wheezes of the asthmatic or the murmur of the worst heart defects muffled and unrecognizable. It is the same for all of the medical students, and I think about all the things about which I had been so wrong. They will need a library, electricity, blood cultures, and a CT scanner someday. But even before this progress is made and despite the chaos around them, they need to listen to their patients. They need to listen not only to the hearts and lungs but to their words, spoken and unspoken, just the same. The students are tired and they are overworked, but it is not enough to simply write out a prescription for quinine to every febrile child. They must not forget that even in the absence of lecturers, books, and laboratory tests, their patients are still the most important teachers of all. I realize as I leave the ward that nothing perceptible has changed. The rusting metal cribs are still full of febrile toddlers receiving quinine infusions and asthmatics underdosed on their inhaled medications who will be discharged wheezing as furiously as they were when they arrived. Looking down the length of the room, I feel as if I should be more disappointed at my overwhelming lack of impact, but instead I find myself resigned.

Before I finally go, Trokon, Robert, and Yatta tell me that maybe they will become pediatricians if the hospital can find a way to train them. They thank me for my morning lectures and my help preparing for their exams. They are only being polite, but I allow myself to be pleased. I realize that this role as teacher and colleague should have been the one I aimed for all along.

In Liberia, things are slowly getting better. I almost envy these doctors' place in history, of how they will be able to look back on their careers and know that they did the work that others did not have the strength to do and that their country is a healthier place because of them. I leave Trokon the stethoscope I had been given upon entering medical school, and I know that he will use it well.

Epilogue

Before I can agree to have a baby, Daryl and I take one last trip. If all goes well, this will be our final chance to move around freely, unencumbered, in places where the mosquitoes could carry malaria and the water might not be clean. My senior year of residency is somehow slipping by quickly. The months on the calendar I had blocked off in red to illustrate for Daryl when we could not start trying were suddenly past. So we buy plane tickets to Sri Lanka, where my college friend Emily is working for the State Department and we can enjoy unlimited government-funded air conditioning. I leave first, ostensibly to do some work that will justify the trip as an "elective." Then several weeks later, Daryl arrives. We make a wide loop across the island, carefully avoiding the north where the Tamil Tigers are still fighting. During those two weeks, we stand in the cool damp air of the rock temples at Dambulla and climb Sigiriya, the hardened magma remains at the center of a volcanic cone that had long since washed away. We swim in the midst of schools of brightly colored damsel and banner fish coral along the atolls of the Maldives. In Unawatuna, a beach town on the southern coast of

Sri Lanka, Daryl loses his wedding band while playing in the surf. He holds his breath and plunges beneath the waves in the place the ring is stripped from his finger, but it is gone, irrevocably lost the moment his hand dragged through and was caught against the gritty sand.

We comb the beach for hours. Long after the light has started to fail, we walk beside each other and I do not look up to meet his face. My eyes scan the smooth expanse of sand, lingering on small shells or bits of dried kelp, the way the shadows fill in the hollows from which crabs will later emerge. I imagine finding the ring even after Daryl has given up. But it is something I will never be able to deliver. Just as he could not snatch it from the salt water into which it had disappeared, I cannot will the ring back into existence and I cannot take away the loneliness each of us had felt at times over the last two and a half years.

When we return to the States, the residency applicant season is well underway. At both the City Hospital and at Children's, the applicants mill about and chat nervously in their identical dark suits. They hold at their sides leather folders that enclose CVs printed on watermarked 100 percent cotton paper. They have master's degrees in public health, have published impressive papers in scientific journals, or founded grassroots aid agencies for street children in Peru. They all look good in writing and in person, having perfected their résumés and honed their interview skills. But I know that none of this meticulous preparation will actually make any bit of difference. They will arrive in the hospital this coming summer just as scared, just as desperate for affirmation as I had been at the start of my three years of sleepless nights spent walking these halls.

"Choose one thing," they will be told. "There is work and then there is your life outside, but there will not be time for all the things you used to do. That doesn't mean you can't have a hobby, but you have to choose. Pick one thing that you can't live without and do that thing when you're not here. If you don't pick just one thing, then it will always feel as if there isn't time enough."

One thing is not sufficient, I think, with a plate of greasy half-eaten Chinese food balanced on one knee. One thing is not enough to live by. But I cannot tell this to the girl before me, with her uncomfortable-looking heels and her diamond solitaire. I cannot explain to her that to be a resident is to have a disease, to be defined by something outside of your power just as surely as cancer and diabetes and hemophilia have defined, at least for a time, some of the children whom I have been privileged to know. The difference is that residency is something I will leave behind soon enough. I will remain at Children's, true, but as soon as these last few months are finished, I will be able to look forward to sleeping every night in my own bed. I will eat breakfast at home with my husband before I go to work and then at night I will come home again. It is a small thing, almost petty (thinking about it now), but it is the one thing I have most missed.

I think again of Max at times like these, when an overeager applicant asks yet another question I have no way to answer: "Are you happy? Do you ever regret choosing this program?" His face comes to me unbidden, his swollen cheeks raised up to an imaginary sun. There is Grace as well, who by this time has died, and so many others. They do not belong to me alone, but I think of them as mine. They are the part of any day that I do not file away when I walk out the doors of the hospital. I carry them with me wherever I go and I know that they will be joined by many others whom I have not yet met. It would sound morbid if I said this out loud, and the girl across from me would likely make note of the comment on the list that she is assembling of each hospital and would choose to train somewhere else, where the residents are less cynical (or less honest). But it doesn't matter which halls she walks while slipping on her white coat, the story will always be the same.

Shortly after this spring arrives. Stubbornly and after more than one false start, but eventually the tulips push their way up through the cold earth and daffodils dot the green crescents of the Emerald Necklace. It is only a handful of weeks before this academic year, too, will come to an end and we will gather for graduation. I hurry along Longwood on an afternoon off, late (as always) for a choir rehearsal. I am quickly becoming enormously and almost comically pregnant. I am not the only one. In my residency class, Brie, then Kara, then Tamara, then I, then Lara, then Courtney, then Elisha, and finally Cindy will give birth in rapid succession over the course of a handful of months. I was not the only one, it seems, to have my calendar so carefully planned. Though Brie (carrying twins) ended up on prolonged bed rest and the rest of us struggled with the long hours, or had to leave rounds regularly each morning to puke, we came through those nine months more or less unscathed. And the juniors behind us, in looking forward to the same freedoms that we will soon be tasting, sidle up close and in a whisper ask the name of my OB.

It is a time of excitement. While many of us would not physically be going anywhere different, we would all be taking on new jobs and new responsibilities. We would be expected to stand on our own. We would be out in the world caring for children with no one but ourselves to rely on. Lara, just as she had hoped, would leave shortly for the Dominican Republic, where she and her husband, Toby, would work and spend weekends at the beach with little Lucia when she is finally born. Courtney would sign on with the Emergency Department to staff one of their community hospital sites, attending deliveries and stabilizing infants for transport to Children's when they need more advanced care. Leisha, who had stood right beside me each morning as we rounded on Max, would spend an extra year doing research before leaving clinical medicine behind and returning—more or less permanently—to the lab. Our indentures finally finished, we found ourselves contemplating the endless possibilities, the lives we wanted to be living, now that we had the freedom to choose.

But before that happens, we will gather once again and remember what has gone past. Along with the parents and the friends of those who have died, we will lay roses in a great pile at the front of the rows of chairs and speak their names out loud. It is a small gesture, this ceremony, but it is one that many families come back to year after year. There will be music. There will be voices raised in song. I will stand with the choir (a hodgepodge of residents, attendings, and other hospital staff) and sing arrangements of easily recognized pop songs that in any other context I would consider insipid but that somehow—before this sea of faces—bring tears to my eyes. A year ago, when Max's name would have been on the list to be read out solemnly and with great emotion, I did not have the energy to attend. I made excuses. I would be out of town for a wedding or a birthday or an anniversary for some imagined family member or friend. It didn't matter. There was no way I could agree and I did not have the words to explain why.

I eventually regretted my cowardice, but by then it was too late. I had missed Max's parents. I would have liked to have stood with them to tell them that I remembered their son. Certainly they could not be in doubt that he was well loved and missed by those who were close to them. But I wanted to be able to tell them that even I, who knew him for only a short succession of weeks, was moved by his courage and grace. Perhaps this wouldn't have mattered. Perhaps they did not even attend. But then that is all the more reason that I should have been there at the reading of his name.

This year, I am attempting to do better, to make amends. And so I go to every choir rehearsal I can and I agree to the solo they want me to sing. As I look out into the audience, I see that people are crying. Though I risk breaking down myself, I do not look away. I sing, my hands resting lightly on the curve of my stomach, and I wish for these families the same things I wish for my own—a world where contentment and happiness outweigh misery and regret.

I do not cry until later, when the rose ceremony is nearly at an end. The list of names is not brief, and this part of the evening wears on and on. The blossoms that had been offered up in remembrance of each dead child as his or her name is spoken tumble out of the vases in which they have been placed. There is an overwhelming feeling of abundance, despite all the sadness, and there is the scent of roses filling the air. Then a family walks up to the front with an enormous bouquet of sunflowers. I imagine them stopping together, as they must have, at the florist that afternoon. There would be roses, the invitation had said. There was no need to bring flowers, since the hospital would provide them. But Grace had loved sunflowers, her mother once told me. They reminded her of what it felt like to be outside. This was why they always, each day that she was in the hospital, made sure to have two vases full—one on each side of her bed.

Grace's mother and father walk slowly toward the front of the auditorium. Her mother carries the sunflowers while her father keeps one hand lightly resting on the small of his wife's back. They look tired, but no more exhausted than when I last saw them. Grace has, by this time, been gone only a few months. I find myself wondering what would have happened to Sox. Grace's mother presses her face into the round dark center of one perfectly formed sunflower and lets the petals stick to the wetness of her cheeks. Then she holds out her arms, in apology or supplication, and one of the attendants takes the flowers away.

I try to find them when the service has ended, but by the time the crowd has thinned out enough for me to push my way to an exit, they are gone. The sun is setting and the crowd tumbles out into the warm spring air, balancing bottled drinks and cafeteria brownies.

On the grass outside the auditorium, children are playing—children who are well, who skip and hop and scrape knees and rush to be scooped up in waiting arms. They are the reason behind it all, the glimmer of hope and of transcendence, the promise that one day there will not be any that can't be saved.

Inside my own belly I can feel that assurance of new beginnings, the small life squirming inside a space too small for it, moving closer to freedom with each liquid breath. Even after it has become familiar, the sensation still brings with it the sharp intake of air that makes me pause with a hand laid flat over my expanding midsection, expecting at any moment that the fluttering will stop and not return again in the ensuing hours or days. Even after multiple ultrasounds, I am half convinced that I am pregnant only in my imagination, that it is not possible that I have come this far. Just as three years earlier I had become a doctor only by painful repetition, by the snapping open of a laryngoscope or the gentle pressure of two fingers searching for a pulse, in the months I have before me I will become something else as well. They say you become a mother the moment the slick infant is placed into your arms, but I know that this isn't true. That isn't how I became a pediatrician and I don't expect that parenting should be any less deliberate or arrived at any easier than this other, tentative confidence I've gained. It is right that such things, such identities, take time. They should be worked at and thought over carefully—savored, like whispered conversations between two friends or red wine tickling the edges of the tongue.

It will happen gradually then, this next transition, just as all things that are good and worth waiting for occur. There will be the forty or so weeks and then the delivery, and then there will be all that comes after. Contained within this promise will be so much more than that first moment of wet skin held tight against my chest or what follows from it, the feedings and diaper changes and the fitful naps that do not ever really give full rest. They tell me to prepare myself, the parents I meet in parks or on street corners or even within the hospital, for the lack of sleep that I have ahead. But I have been tired before. I have emerged dazed but determined, and I am not afraid. I feel the weariness deep inside me as I have felt before, but this time it brings with it an excitement I can barely contain within my ever-growing form. There will be time for sleep when all this has finished. And there will be time for all other things as well.

About the Author

Meghan MacLean Weir, MD, obtained her undergraduate degree at Princeton University majoring in molecular biology with work on viral protein expression, then went on to study medicine at Stony Brook University. She was also awarded an MSc degree in Medical Anthropology from the Institute for Social and Cultural Anthropology at Oxford University for work done there on the impact of poverty, undernutrition, and infections on children in sub-Saharan Africa. She completed her residency training in pediatrics at Children's Hospital Boston and Boston Medical Center; during this time she held the position of teaching fellow in pediatrics at the Boston University School of Medicine and clinical fellow in pediatrics at the Harvard Medical School. She has participated in research and training programs in South Africa, Liberia, and Sri Lanka that have been funded in part by the Stony Brook School of Medicine, Children's Hospital Boston, Massachusetts General Hospital, and the American Academy of Pediatrics. Her essays have appeared in hospital publications at both her former and current institutions, and excerpts of her writing have been used in the Humanism in Medicine curriculum for interns at the Boston Combined Residency Program. She and her family live in the Boston area, where she works as a pediatrician in the Emergency departments of Boston Children's and Beverly Hospitals.

Printed in the United States
By Bookmasters